'Cuts through all the beauty fluff.'
FARRAH STORR, ELLE

INSTYLE
BEST BEAUTY BOOK

COSMOPOLITAN
BEST BOOK

'Your new beauty bible.'
COSMOPOLITAN

'Expert advice.'
THE SUN

'Must Read'
BEST MAGAZINE

'Get the book club on to… *Great Skin.*'
EVENING STANDARD

GREAT SKIN

SECRETS THE BEAUTY INDUSTRY DOESN'T TELL YOU

Ingeborg van Lotringen

@theogbeautyboss

GIBSON SQUARE

For papa

This edition first published in the USA in 2021 by Gibson Square

ISBN: 978-1-78334-167-2
email: rights@gibsonsquare.com
website: www.gibsonsquare.com

Papers used by Gibson Square are natural, recyclable products made from wood grown in sustainable forests; inks used are vegetable based. Manufacturing conforms to ISO 14001, and is accredited to FSC and PEFC chain of custody schemes. Colour-printing is through a certified CarbonNeutral® company that offsets its CO2 emissions.

CONTENTS

AUTHOR'S NOTE

If you have a skin condition that requires medical assistance, always follow your doctor's advice.

1 GET TO KNOW YOUR SKIN

Test every skincare product and treatment going. That is pretty much my job description as a beauty editor and writer, and has been for more than two decades. When I tell people this, they often ask two questions—what are the Best Products Ever? And, what are the Miracle Treatments I swear by? These questions always make me break out in a cold sweat. In an age of bite-size advice and 'gurus' speaking in certainties, I get that we expect fail-safe routes to great skin. But it is also nonsense, in my experience. There are no magic bullets in skincare.

Not only do we all have different skin types and genes, our skin is also influenced by the seasons, diet, health, stress levels, hormones, the environment (life, basically). Despite being 'only cosmetics', skincare affects a living organ that's unique and constantly changing in its needs. The best products for me aren't automatically the best products for you. The best products for you in the summer may not be the best in winter, or on a sunny holiday, or in the city.

In order to know what is right for you, you first of all have to get to know that amazing surface organ of your body better. You don't have to be a skin expert for this. I am a journalist and not a scientist, doctor or beautician. But I touch and see my skin every day and know more about its fluctuating quirks than any one expert ever could. Also, I have got to know more about it through the knowledge gathered over the years from dermatologists, plastic surgeons, scientists, and other skin professionals. And so can you.

Once you know your skin, step two is learning just how choose from the overwhelming number of potions on offer. This book is meant to help you expand what you know about your own skin in fifty ways and insights so that your choice of products will be based on what is good for *your* skin, not on what anyone with a nice glow (real or Facetuned) happens to rate as the Best Ever.

The chapters in this book are based on innumerable questions readers have shared with me about their concerns and on over two decades of personal and professional experience receiving, testing and researching the skincare that is sent to me by countless brands. Yes, it's a perk of the job, but as you will find out, it can also be quite the pitfall.

As a journalist, I like to get to the bottom of things and I have dedicated hundreds and hundreds of hours to interviewing the global-beauty industry's brightest minds whom I have been lucky enough to meet regularly. More than that, these meetings and exchanges have fostered ongoing conversations about the precise details of skincare. Having picked (and picked again) so many of these lab-based and skin-obsessed brains and having read their books, papers and references, I have learned what's possible and achievable and can see when promising new directions develop.

But for the real proof that the power of skincare is

based on self-knowledge, I merely have to point to my beauty-team colleagues at the magazines I worked for as a beauty director. The ones who arrived with problem-free skin maintained and refined it, and the passing of time has made little difference. The ones who struggled with breakouts, rosacea, or acne got their issues under control within months of immersing themselves in the logic of skincare, and today have skin they are proud of. Getting to know our skin is a by-product of our job as beauty writers. Instead of falling for the latest prettiest advertising picture or most tempting slogan, we start to look out for the right products for our skin and learn to find them and stick with them.

There are not enough jobs as a beauty journalist to go round for everyone, unfortunately! But I have aimed to distil in this book all or most of what you would discover. What is in these chapters is not quite as simple as scoring a list of solutions. Nonetheless, it's doable stuff. Spending quality time with your skin will make it a cinch to select the best products for you from the many thousands on offer. That goes for skin of every colour, incidentally, because the rules are the same—most of the time. When they're not I will point out the differences and alternative approaches.

My dad gave me good skin—so yes, luck and genes also play a role. But I still had to find ways to honour that gift so as not to squander it. At the same time, the right products can make a massive difference to what Mother Nature gave you, making it possible to learn how to change your skin's fortunes, whatever state it's in.

It will require some patience. Most products take a good two months to start showing real results. So, unless you experience irritation or discomfort (which almost always means you should stop using it), stick with a product for at least this amount of time. Chopping and changing is not going help the good health of your skin.

You will come across cryptic-looking ingredient names along the way. But don't let that put you off. I could describe both a pot of cold cream and a *hyaluronic acid* serum as 'moisturiser' to make things look plain and simple. But it would not be very helpful to you. Blame chemists and Latin-loving botanists for the jargon, but delving a little bit deeper can mean the difference between finding a good product or buying a nonsense one. Even if some of the ingredients' names look like identical twins, you'll discover that their number is actually quite manageable. Soon your skin will reward you, too, for the effort.

I have added in many chapters products I like as examples (listed from inexpensive to treat-yourself territory). But they are just starting points. After reading this book, you'll be so clued up on skincare that you'll want to seek out the very best products for yourself.

* PART ONE *

YOUR ROUTINE

While there are no magic bullets in skincare, there are a number of things that create the baseline you'll need. It is the blank canvas against which you can get to know your skin and its needs. They consist of two things, routine and what I will call 'gold standards' in the text. The bad news about the routine is that some of it is stuff you should start doing, well, yesterday, to be honest. The good news is that it doesn't take much time or money.

2 A SKINCARE REGIME

TRY IT, IT ACTUALLY WORKS

Given the billions we spend on the stuff, 'does skincare really work?' is an odd question. But it is a good one. If you were to ask a general practitioner for non-medical advice on skincare they would likely say, 'you may as well put some E45 on it'. Then you meet someone with great skin who appears to have looked after it with a lot more than just a lick of cold cream and you wonder how they did it. So you pinball between trusting the promises made by beauty brands and resigning yourself to the point of view that skincare is at most a bit of hydration.

It gets worse. All beauty and medical professionals keenly agree that cosmetics are *not* medicine. In fact, the definition of a cosmetic is so disheartening, you might well be tempted to stick to cold cream for life after reading it. Cosmetics-industry body CTPA says, 'a cosmetic is meant to perfume or temporarily enhance the appearance, and cannot modify the way skin or hair functions. If it does, it should be classed as a medicine and prescribed by a doctor.' Off-the-shelf and over-the-counter skincare falls under this definition, as does 'professional' skincare (as sold in cosmetic clinics) and 'cosmeceutical' skincare, supposedly a hybrid between a cosmetic and medicine but really an unregulated term invented by the cosmetic industry.

The US Food and Drug Administration (FDA) will categorise cosmetics as drugs if they are 'articles intended for use in the diagnosis, cure, mitigation, treatment, or prevention of disease' and products '(other than food) intended to affect the structure or any function of the body of man'. It means, for example, that a dandruff shampoo, fluoride toothpaste, or cellulite cream will require FDA certification because the product has a therapeutic effect. If no approval is needed, it means the product is merely 'intended to be rubbed, poured, sprinkled, or sprayed on, introduced into, or otherwise applied to the human body... for cleansing, beautifying, promoting attractiveness, or altering the appearance'.

All this certainly gives the impression that we are idiots for putting our faith and money into any of it. And indeed, often we are. If a product is mostly water and mineral oil (like, er, cold cream), plus lots of preservatives and inert fillers, with miniscule percentages of active ingredients or botanicals, paying more than a quid or two for a jar would make you a bit of a numpty.

Nor is that easy to avoid for any of us. The world's $500-plus-billion cosmetic industry has to list every ingredient a product contains in order of volume on the packaging in what is called the INCI (International Nomenclature of Cosmetic Ingredients) list. But that's about all it's required to do by way of transparency. Brands don't have to disclose just how much of each ingredient is included, or whether or not it's at a proven active level, or whether it is in a formula that can actually have an effect on your skin. Meanwhile, brands are perfectly within their right to make a big (big) play of what their ingredients, under ideal circumstances and at active levels, have been proven to do. What they don't have to do is spell out whether this is also true for the particular formula they are selling.

At the other end of the cosmetic spectrum are the brands that can provide both clinical proof of their ingredients' effectiveness and that of their product formulas. But they will want to underplay their promises to an extent. If their product's claims go beyond the function of a cosmetic, it could well run the risk of being classed a prescription-only drug and be shut out of the lucrative cosmetics market.

No wonder that a semi-scientific universe of unverified claims, nebulous promises, and skewed terminology ('brightens the appearance of the skin') has mushroomed. You can never be quite sure whether a cosmetic does what it says on the tin or whether it is closer to snake oil. No wonder that everyone is confused and skincare sometimes gets a bad rap.

The body doesn't prioritise fighting a rash, dis-colouration, wrinkles, patches, redness, acne, oiliness etc. visible on the outside. Skin may be our largest organ, but when it comes to the nutrients we ingest, skin gets the dregs of everything after other organs have been seen to.

But good cosmetic ingredients deliver nutrients and hydration directly where they are required. They provide skin with the essential tools for being healthy all over, without bumps and spots, keeping them at bay for the future. The cosmetic industry is a phenomenal resource for tackling skincare concerns and constantly spends money on research to provide the consumer with the tools to do so.

Notwithstanding the CTPA's modest definition of a cosmetic, the fact is that plenty of skincare is active to the point where it will change and improve your skin long-term. For example, in the US the cosmeceutical brand iS Clinical supplies a number of cancer hospitals with a selection of its formulas, including its Poly Vitamin Serum and Pro Heal Serum Advance+. The reason? These products help heal and regenerate skin compromised by radio or chemotherapy, a fact observed and acknowledged by oncologists.

So, good skincare does work. You just need to know which products, ingredients and brands to pick and how to decipher their contents. In the case of cosmeceuticals, one way of finding out whether you are dealing with an effective one is to check whether the product website provides independent clinical trials on its formulations.

Of course, our skin's requirements can vary so much from one person to the next and one season to the next, that a product that performs near 'miracles' on one person's skin may do nothing, or worse, could aggravate, someone else's. But by the end of this book, you'll be able to navigate your way through standing on your head.

It means that you will need a basic knowledge of which ingredients are active helpers, and which are not, as well as an understanding of what your skin needs at a particular moment in time. Otherwise all you can do is accept that your purchase is the equivalent of an (often expensive) lottery ticket. Or that you'll just have to wait, say, until the beauty industry adopts the type of detailed information pharmaceutical companies are obliged to enclose with medication. Like never.

BOTTOM LINE: GOOD COSMETICS CAN DO A LOT

3 SKIN TYPE

IT ISN'T EVERYTHING

The first step in your own skincare regime is to know your basic skin type. There are generally four skin types: *dry, oily, combination* and *normal*. Sensitive skin is not a skin type, it's a condition brought on by extrinsic (environmental) factors.

You're born with your skin type, but that doesn't mean you have to put up with its characteristics: the right skincare and lifestyle choices can seriously improve how your skin behaves. Get it right consistently, and dry, oily or combination skin may reward you by acting more like holy-grail 'normal' skin in the long run.

The classic way to determine your skin type is by washing your face. Use a mild, sulphate-free face wash and wait 20 minutes without putting anything else on your face. If, at this point, your face feels or looks:

Tight, arid, sometimes flaky (in fact, your skin will feel like this all the time, all over your body): you have dry skin (more later, but your skin lacks lipids and you need nourishing products rich in oils and skin-barrier-repairing lipids). *If these symptoms come and go, however, or are evident on your face but nowhere else on your body, your skin may be dehydrated (lacking in water), which is a skin condition and not a skin type. Water-rich moisturisers rich in humectants are your first port of call.*

Shiny and a bit slick with large pores: you have oily skin (more on this later, but try pore-clearing *salicylic acid* and water-based hydrating serums).

Shiny in the middle (T-Zone), dry and tight on the cheeks: this is combination skin (more on this later, but try water-based hydration all over, with a richer lipid-restoring cream where needed, and balancing ingredients like *niacinamide*.

Smooth, glowing and comfortable: congratulations, this is normal skin. (You will keep it if you give your skin normal daily care and protection.)

You'll find plenty of advice on the right (and wrong) ingredients, textures, and products for your skin type as you work your way through this book. Of course, many (though hardly all) products will tell you what skin type they're meant to be for, but I'd like to caution you to always scan the INCI list on the back of the pot as well. There are brands that get skin types exactly right (Paula's Choice is one of them). But I also see plenty of 'oily skin' products full of alcohol, or creams for 'delicate, dry' skins with fragrance and other irritants, and 'combination skin' products that strip instead of balance.

BOTTOM LINE: BUYING PRODUCTS MARKED FOR YOUR SKIN TYPE ISN'T A FAIL-SAFE STRATEGY

4 GOLD STANDARD: CLEANSING

YOU MUST CLEANSE, HERE'S WHY

The first thing to do to get to know your skin is to guide it to a neutral position where it is not stressed out. And that first and foremost means daily cleansing. A friend once decided to stop washing or cleaning his face for several months. This would, he insisted, teach his skin to 'self-cleanse', which supposedly was its 'natural state'. Our use of soaps and other unnecessary cosmetics just got in the way.

It wasn't a new idea as far as I was concerned. Just a dumb one. Within a few weeks, he was scratching his itching face, which looked raw in places and oily in others. His complexion turned blotchy and he developed a form of adult acne, along with eczema. The experiment ended pretty quickly.

Funnily enough, whoever told him about the 'dangers' of soap had a point. Most bar soaps and the majority of liquid soaps are based on detergents that, along with dirt and excess sebum, will strip away skin's lipid layer, or acid mantle. It's a veil of beneficial skin lipids and delicately balanced 'good' and 'bad' bacteria (called the skin microbiome) whose job it is to keep moisture inside the skin and invaders, such as too many disease-causing bacteria and free radicals, out.

The acid mantle will recover after a few hours, but it's vulnerable while scrambling to re-assemble itself. If you keep going at your skin with the wrong cleansers for long enough, its self-repair system will falter and cracks will start showing in skin's bacterial acid/lipid armour. The result? Inflammation, oily breakouts, acne, redness, eczema—basically, anything that constitutes a 'problem skin'.

So what went wrong with our soap dodger? He took a good principle, misunderstood it, and went way overboard with it. Not cleansing is as bad as bad cleansing. Left with too many dead surface cells, excess oil and all the filth and pollution that gets stuck to them in a modern city, pores will clog and the system will be under nonstop attack from its surface. Grime creates its own cell and acid mantle-destroying invaders, so soap dodgers end up with the same problems as those of soap fiends.

Some still maintain that our skin is so finely tuned that it could balance itself out if left well enough (and long enough) alone. And well it might if you lived in an oxygen bubble without UV, pollution, dirt, fumes, stress, and basically anything that comes with modern living in the real world. That grandma who used 'nothing but soap and water her whole life and had the best skin' (everybody seems to have heard of one) may have lived a relatively stress-free life in the countryside in a moderate climate. And if that's your skin, too, congratulations and good luck with your soap. If not, skip the bar soap and water, particularly when washing your face.

BOTTOM LINE: OUR SKIN DOESN'T SELF-CLEANSE

5 DOUBLE-CLEANSING

IT IS NOT A NONSENSE

So, if not bar soap and water, then what? The answer is cleansing twice in a row at night (in the morning, once is fine) with the right products. This is not a waste of time and money. Why? Because makeup, sebum (the stuff your skin produces to lubricate itself), sweat, dust, grime and toxic particulate matter make for a cocktail that settles at different levels of depth on your skin and inside your pores.

A quick splash of water will dissolve none of it, and a perfunctory wash won't cut it either, for some elements of this filth cake are oil-soluble and others water-soluble.

So, for me, the best way to cleanse gently and

thoroughly is to use an oil or cream cleanser first, massaged into the face for 30 seconds or so and rinsed or tissued or muslin-clothed off. Follow that with a foamy face wash or gel to eek out any water-soluble pollutants and rinse away any excess oil. And that should do it. With the right products, this will:

* Get rid of your eye makeup along with everything else (if anything is left, a little bi-phase eye makeup remover—of the type you shake before use—on a cotton pad will soak it off in seconds).

* Cost you no more than single-cleansing because you need only a little of each cleanser.

* Leave skin entirely clean but never dry or tight-feeling—because you've got rid of the dirt but not the skin's lipid barrier or acid mantle.

* Make serums and creams effective. Put those on un-cleansed skin and they'll just slide off your clogged pores. Skincare actives have a job penetrating deep enough into the

skin at the best of times; what chance have they got when the canvas isn't even clean?

Some people make a whole wash-basin 'ritual' of this, which is nice when you have the time and the inclination. But cleansing is such an important daily habit that it ought to be quick and easy—so personally, I just do my double-cleansing in the shower. One caveat here: hot water dries skin out, so I try to make sure the water I splash in my face is cool enough.

If you are totally wedded to your oil-based or water-based cleanser, you can use the same cleanser twice if you like, instead of two different ones. And on makeup-free or away-from-the-city days, even a double-cleanse drill sergeant like me will (sometimes) ditch the second go.

The most important thing is that you don't skip cleansing altogether, no matter how fetching you think that rock chick-eye looks in the morning. It just means doing your skin a massive disservice, and setting it up for future problems.

Micellar water

Despite the hype that hailed them as the Second Coming of cleansers, micellar waters (the peculiar name itself makes them sound important) do not replace the need for double cleansing. Soaked into a cotton pad and swiped across the skin, they are often, misleadingly, described as 'waters infused with tiny oil droplets that attract dirt like magnets'. The suggestion is not only that this is an ultra-gentle way to cleanse, but also that it is quick and convenient as it's a no-rinse method.

The truth is that the 'oil droplets' (or *'micelles'*—it's a French invention), suspended in the water base are tiny clusters of oil and surfactants (cleansing agents). They work together, with the oil bit attracting sebum and dirt and the surfactant lifting the lot off the skin.

The fact that the oil does half the work allows, in most (but not all) cases, for the surfactant to be mild and non-stripping. But you still don't want to leave the micellar liquid on your face, so you should rinse it off with water.

So although it's effective (it gets rid of eye makeup as well) and usually gentle, micellar water is no single-step substitute for your double-cleansing regime. Use it to remove most of your makeup, then follow it with an oil or water-based rinse-off cleanser. Either type is fine.

Cleansing wipes

If you must use them, only get biodegradable or compostable cleansing wipes (and even then, only ever bin rather than flush them). Only use them in exceptional circumstances if no alternative is readily available. More often than not they contain strong detergents, alcohol and other drying, irritating agents (it makes no difference whether they are called organic) and their residue should be rinsed off. But that is very unlikely to happen if they are your 'bedside staple'. So it's best to avoid bad habits altogether. Your skin will reward you.

BOTTOM LINE: DON'T GO TO BED WITHOUT CLEANSING YOUR FACE

6 AVOID SULPHATES

YOU NEED TO GO SULPHATE-FREE

Sulphates are foamy detergents one finds in washing up liquid, washing powder, car wash, bubble bath and, oh, face cleansers. The cheapest and most popular for personal care products are *sodium lauryl sulphate* and *sodium laureth sulphate* (SLS and SLES respectively, but often grouped together as SLS). But there are lots of other sulphates: *TEA-lauryl sulphate*, *magnesium lauryl sulphate*, *sodium coco sulphate*, the list goes on.

Sulphates cut through grease like Fairy Liquid, and create fabulous clouds of bubbles. They also rip the lipids off your skin and disrupt its protective acid mantle as they are alkaline—the opposite of acidic.

They're not toxic, deadly or carcinogenic, they're just good at causing long-term dryness and irritation. For your body, anything ending in *sulphate* is almost as stripping as alcohol (with *sodium lauryl* and *sodium laureth sulphate* being the worst of the bunch).

The simple message is that you don't want these in your face wash, body cleanser, or, as far as I'm concerned, shampoo. Many brands will shout 'no SLS' all over their packaging but, to be honest, pretty much none of the sulphates mentioned are top choices, especially for your face.

As for the bubbles sulphates are so good at creating, here's an interesting fact. In themselves they have no cleansing ability whatsoever. We've just been conditioned, through a century of 'creamy soap lather' and particularly laundry detergent ads, to associate lots of suds with cleanliness.

But your skin is a living thing and not a piece of

clothing. Whether your cleanser produces a bath full of bubbles or no more than a fine foam has no bearing on how well it will clean the skin. However, it can be quite a good indication that it has just removed your skin's acid mantle.

While lots of bubbles don't equal cleanliness, it doesn't mean all foamy detergents are the devil's spawn, either. Dozens of mild detergents that don't strip skin have been developed over the years, many of which create perfectly nice suds on your skin. Furthermore, when you rub these in for at least twenty seconds, the bubbles will help remove viruses. So if you don't feel clean without bubbles, there is no need to go without them.

Ingredients ending with the word *glucoside*, *glutamate*, *taurate* or *sulfosuccinate* are examples of gentle foamy detergents, while those ending with *betaine* are generally gentle enough. Just check the INCI list on your cleanser for these.

BOTTOM LINE: SULPHATES SHOULD NOT GO ANYWHERE NEAR YOUR FACE

Sulphate-free cleansers whose ingredients I like:
Garnier Micellar Water Sensitive Skin
YourGoodSkin Revitalizing Foaming Wash
Mother Dirt Cleanser For Face And Body
Dr Sam's Flawless Cleanser

7 AND SKIP BAR SOAP AS WELL

So, if *sulphates* are as bad as all that, is the good old bar soap the better choice of face cleanser, particularly if 'superfatted' with rich plant oils?

Well no. To make a block of soap, its fatty ingredients have to be 'saponified', that is, mixed with caustic soda (*sodium hydroxide*), which is a highly alkaline, industrial-strength chemical. At home you'll find it in drain cleaner in your kitchen-sink cabinet. It doesn't make soap dangerous as the caustic soda mostly evaporates. But the resulting soap is still alkaline like SLS and other sulphates. On our mildly-acidic skin this is irritating and drying, no matter how much shea butter you pack into the bar of soap.

And what of all those new 'cleansing bars' that are, apparently, not soap, but just look like it? Dove was among the first to make one of these 'syndets': bars not made of saponified oils, but mild synthetic detergents. Though touted as a gentle alternative to soap, they generally don't use the very mildest detergents (I've spotted shampoo bars that were basically solid SLS).

As a rule of thumb, I would still recommend a *sulphate*-free face wash or a cleansing oil over a syndet, particularly if you are starting out on finding the double-cleansing regime that establishes the neutral state of your skin.

Nonetheless, some recent arrivals, by brands such as Drunk Elephant, Sebamed and Gallinée, have been making great leaps forward. Their bars are so mild they are akin to a non-stripping face wash.

Look for the words 'soap-free' and 'cleansing bar' rather than anything that calls itself 'soap'. Also look for a mention of the pH on the packaging to check whether the syndet is acidic.

Our skin has a pH between 4.7 to 5.5 and the syndet should be between 5.5 and 6.5 (the lower, the better).

BOTTOM LINE: BAR SOAPS ARE A BAD CHOICE FOR YOUR FACE

Syndets whose ingredients I like:

Sebamed Cleansing Bar for Sensitive and Problematic Skin

Gallinée Cleansing Bar

8 CLEANSING OILS

NOT ALL OF THEM ARE CREATED EQUAL

Because the skin is a living organ, cleansing it is rather different from cleaning an object. For example, it means that oils can be great for cleansing your skin. They dissolve sebum (the lipidic coating our skin produces) and dislodge dirt.

Especially if you have oily skin (meaning it over-produces sebum, causing spots and oiliness), the idea may sound counter-intuitive and I know plenty of people with an oily skin who have no intention of ever using a cleansing oil (nor should you feel you have to use oils to cleanse). But others who switch to cleansing oil or 'balm' (which is oil-based) never look back.

Once you get over tackling oil with oil, you'll find

that the right oil cleanser not only leaves skin clean, it conditions it as well, thanks to (non-greasy) fatty acids for your skin's acid mantle—they can leave dry skin supple and make oily skin less prone to breakouts.

That's if you stick certain (plant) oils such as *squalane, jojoba oil* and *rosehip oil*. Not every oil is the same.

Mineral oils can be found on your INCI list as *paraffinum liquidum*, *petrolatum*, *paraffin oil*. Despite the word 'mineral', they have nothing to do with essential minerals (good for your health) and mineral makeup (good for your skin). They're purified petroleum by-products that are inert.

That means mineral oils have no active molecules—plant oils do have these—and are unlikely to irritate, but also that they have no conditioning properties. (In moisturisers, their sole function is to form a layer on the skin's surface that stops moisture from evaporating.)

Although they are, despite what you might have

read, low on the list of pore-clogging (comedogenic) ingredients, they're still not a great option for oily skin. A high dose of them could leave you with breakouts instead of preventing them.

Unfortunately, the plant oils I mentioned are expensive while mineral oils, and other synthetic oils (such as *isopropyl myristate*, which is also said to be the main ingredient in anti-corrosion solvent WD40 and can clog pores when used in large quantities) cost practically nothing. Not surprising-ly, the latter two often end up in cleansing balms or oils to keep the price down.

The good news is that there are low-cost synthesised but plant-derived oils that are good for every skin. So a good oil-based cleanser does not need to be expensive. An example is *caprylic triglyc-eride* (made from glycerin and coconut or palm kernel fatty acids).

These cleansers needn't feel greasy either. Most cleansing balms and oils contain a small amount of emulsifier, or mild surfactant, that make the oil turn to milk on contact with water, helping the stuff rinse clean off.

It means you need to massage your oil onto dry skin to allow it to do its dirt-dissolving job; only then do you emulsify the whole lot with water and let it wash down the plughole.

Before you decide to save some money and source your cleansing oil from the kitchen cabinet—these oils obviously won't contain emulsifiers so won't come off particularly easily. Plus some, like *olive oil*, can be very irritating, while others are ace at clogging pores. *Coconut, palm* and *flaxseed oil,* as well as *cocoa butter*, are some of the biggest comedogenic offenders.

BOTTOM LINE: A PLANT-BASED CLEANSING OIL IS WORTH TRYING, EVEN IF YOU HAVE OILY SKIN

Cleansing oils and balms whose ingredients I like:
The Body Shop Camomile Silky Cleansing Oil
Pai Light Work Rosehip Cleansing Oil
Merumaya Melting Cleansing Balm
Time Bomb Peace & Quiet Cleansing Oil
Clinique Take The Day Off Cleansing Balm

9 OILINESS

ADD THE RIGHT PORE-UNPLUGGER

If you're prone to oiliness and spots, or are going through a spell of them, then your daily cleanser should have *salicylic acid* in it. It doesn't only unblock and de-gunk pores, it's antibacterial and anti-inflammatory, so it calms as it clears, which is really important. A little of it every day will balance your skin and is likely to make a difference within weeks.

Tea tree oil is another popular pore-clearing ingredient with decent anti-microbial properties. Astringent (pore-contracting) *witch hazel* is another, but it tends to come in an alcohol distillation and that alcohol means the cleanser will cause more problems than it solves.

This is a good moment to talk about *alcohol* as an ingredient. *Alcohol* may annihilate oil slicks on your skin and satisfyingly bite into spots, but both will come back with a vengeance not long after you have subjected your skin to too much of it. It strips and inflames the skin, which are precisely some of the factors that cause acne.

So if you see *SD alcohol, isopropyl alcohol, ethyl alcohol, ethanol*, or *alcohol denat.* featured high on the INCI list, avoid the product altogether. And I don't just mean in cleansers: in *any* skincare. As a rule of thumb, if you can smell alcohol when putting a product on your skin, buy something else. It will generally do more harm than good.

But don't go mad. Unlike anything with the word *sulphate*, not everything with the word '*alcohol*' is to be avoided. *Cetearyl, stearyl,* and *cetyl alcohol* are fatty alcohols that serve as emulsifiers and are harmless. *Benzyl alcohol*, meanwhile, is used as a preservative that's fine for your skin in low doses. Just check that it is near the bottom of the INCI list.

BOTTOM LINE: SALICYLIC ACID WILL SUBDUE SPOTS, ALCOHOL CAN MAKE THEM WORSE

Pore-purifying cleansers whose ingredients I like:

The Inkey List Salicylic Acid Cleanser

CeraVe SA Smoothing Cleanser

Vichy Normaderm Phytosolution Cleansing Gel

10 CLEANSING BRUSHES

RISKY BUSINESS

The effects of a mechanical cleansing brush can be a revelation, literally. Dull, congested skin will emerge smoother and brighter with repeated use, thanks to layers of encrusted dead cells being got rid of and the brush action bringing roses to your cheeks (that's blood circulation being revved up).

It's no wonder, then, that those new to decent cleansing develop a bit of a reliance on their buzzing friends.

And that's a problem. Once the dead cells are gone, your cleansing brush will start aggravating the healthy ones. Skin is always turning over, so some people maintain there are always dead cells to tackle, but in the same way that you wouldn't use a foot file every day, your face needs a regular break from sloughing as well.

I wouldn't use a cleansing brush more than twice a week. If I used one at all, I would choose the gentlest model marketed for sensitive skin (even if I didn't have sensitive skin). I would use it for its ability to get rid of big-city toxic residues better than regular cleansing methods, but if I lived in the countryside breathing uncongested air, there would be no point.

But, and here comes the biggest worry I have, I would do the above only if I knew I was meticulous about keeping my bathroom and all my make-up gadgets spotless and disinfected, which I'm not.

The problem with cleansing brushes is that they become fertile breeding grounds for moulds and unpleasant bacteria in the hands of anyone but the most fastidious germophobes. Silicone-nibbed cleansing devices, such as the Foreo, don't have that issue and are less abrasive to boot, so are probably the better option if you're truly intent on using mechanical cleansing every day.

In that case I would never double up and use it alongside a face scrub—only one or the other. Combining your mechanical cleanser with an acid cleanser is another case of doubling up, while a definite 'do' is to use them with a gentle cleanser of your own choice. The cleansers sold alongside the brushes are usually best avoided.

BOTTOM LINE: A CLEANSING BRUSH IS NOT AN ESSENTIAL PART OF ANYONE'S SKINCARE REGIME

11 THE FUNCTION OF TONERS

THEY ARE MUCH MISUNDERSTOOD

The 'cleanse, tone, moisturise' adage has been hammered into us for generations. But, judging from the questions I get, nobody really understands *why* they need to use a toner, most simply think that they *should*. For decades the majority of toners were basically alcohol solutions that dissolved cleansing milk residue or 'treated oiliness'. I still have a bottle of Clean & Clear Lotion that I won't let anywhere near my face. I do, however, use it to disinfect tweezers and nail clippers.

Alternative toners based on ingredients like *rosewater* and *witch hazel* instead of alcohol could be classed as less offensive, but as so many modern cleansers are wash-off and leave no residue, what is the point?

Well, it seems there might be a very good one. 'New' toners (the type has in fact been around forever, it just got mostly forgotten), aim to re-balance skin's pH. Every part of our body has its own optimum pH level to help it thrive, and skin's comfort zone is between 4.7 and 5.5. This is the 'acid mantle' that protects the skin that I've mentioned before (and will again many times).

Cleansing, even if you use the mildest surfactant, can throw off this acidic pH, temporarily increasing it to over 5.5 and making it prone to dryness and irritation. This is even the case if you use just water. Water has a neutral (meaning it sits smack between acidic and alkaline) pH of 7, and in hard-water areas can even be slightly alkaline. So it's always less acidic than skin, explaining that mildly dry feeling you get after the water you've splashed on your face dries up.

Your toner will come to the rescue. The new, quick-penetrating liquid toners with ingredients such as *prebiotics, lactic acid*, anti-inflammatories and *glycerine* are the fastest way to restore skin to a state of calm, balance, hydration and an optimum receptiveness to further skincare ingredients.

You can wipe them on with a saturated cotton pad (lifting more oils and residue in the process) or simply splash them on your face. Sometimes they are sold in a mist and can also be used to fix your skin's moisture levels and pH throughout the day. I decant my favourite toner in a spray bottle.

These new toners are pretty versatile, as are the ways they are marketed. They can go by the name of toner, tonic, lotion, softener or even face vinegar. Which can be pretty confusing. So make sure you check the INCI list for a mix of the ingredients mentioned earlier, while avoiding alcohol.

Don't reach for 'acid' or 'brightening' toners. Such products are essentially acid-based liquid peels and not toners. You will find out more about peels later.

BOTTOM LINE: MODERN TONERS ARE A VERSATILE SKIN TREAT

Toners whose ingredients I like
Simple Kind to Skin Soothing Facial Toner
Gallinée Face Vinegar
Origins Essence Lotion With Dual Ferment Complex
Estée Lauder Micro Essence Skin Activating Treatment
     Lotion

12 GOLD STANDARD: MOISTURIS-ING

NOT THAT COMPLICATED

Is this a minefield? Well it's not literally, obviously. But if you got caught up in the oil-versus-water debate that's been raging among skin experts over the past decade, you might be tempted to give up on moisturiser altogether—and that would be a mistake.

Your skin, whether it's dry or oily, needs irrigation like vegetation to function optimally and look bouncy and translucent. Even very oily skins are often dehydrated, meaning they're lacking water. Drinking the stuff is not enough. Your body will just direct it to other organs first before it (ever) reaches your skin.

And this is where moisturisers come in, featuring a raft of ingredients that infuse, attract and trap water directly where it's needed. Most moisturisers incorporate oils to a greater or lesser extent, their function being partly to keep watery substances from evaporating, and partly to nourish skin with essential lipids, which it needs to stay supple and keep its protective lipid barrier intact.

Some experts take issue with the lipids bit, claiming we make plenty of our own (it's the thing our skin produces called sebum), and that adding them to our skin in the form of creams or face oils would make skin 'lazy' and dial down its auto-lubrication potential.

That may well be true. But it assumes that our skins are always perfectly calibrated machines and not constantly under assault by the environment, hormones and less-than-pure living conditions. All these things have the power to sap oils or send their production haywire. So the question isn't whether moisturiser is 'bad', it's whether your choice of moisturiser is right for the condition your skin is in.

BOTTOM LINE: EVERY SKIN NEEDS SOME LEVEL OF HYDRATION TO LOOK GOOD

13 CHOOSING A MOISTURISER

THINK LIGHT IF IT DOESN'T FEEL TIGHT

Just start with an oil-free moisturiser (technically, we should call it a 'hydrator') and see if your face feels tight at any time during the day. If not, your skin probably produces enough natural lipids to lock in the no-oil hydrators (such as *glycerine, hyaluronic acid* and *polysaccharides*) these gels and lotions are made of, and you're good to go.

If you sense a level of parching as the day wears on, opt for a cream with oils in it, keeping in mind that 'richer' doesn't necessarily equate to 'better' for your skin.

The most efficient, long-lasting moisturisers combine water-attracting 'sponge' ingredients (or humectants) such as *glycerine* with lipids that are already naturally present in the skin, such as *ceramides*, and light-textured oils (emollients) such as *jojoba* and *squalane*; their sebum-like qualities let them penetrate skin and nourish it rather than mostly sitting on top and preventing water loss.

In fact, there is a lot of evidence that those two oils (*jojoba* and *squalane*) in particular can 'trick' oily skin into thinking it's produced enough sebum. Hence they're often called 'balancing' oils. So they could be great even if your skin never feels dry. Whether you want to trial this for two months (the time it takes to assess any skincare's long-term efficiency) is a personal choice; if you simply cannot stand oils, there are good alternative hydrators around to keep you quenched.

If even these creams leave you feeling tight after a few hours, opt for richer, thicker ones targeted at dry skin, featuring 'occlusive' oils and waxes such as *shea butter*, *lanolin* and *argan oil*, or modest levels (meaning, low on the INCI list) of *silicone* and *mineral oil*, that will sit on the skin to keep water from evaporating. But even here, make sure there are also plenty of humectants such as *sorbitol* and *hyaluronic acid* to quench skin, either in the formula or layered under your moisturiser in the form of a serum.

Another thing you can do is add one or two drops of face oil to your daily dollop of not-quite-rich-enough cream right before you apply it.

Less is more though. I found this out the hard way. My skin is normal to dry and I've spent my life buttering it with rich creams just because it felt nice and I could. But recently, while trying to manage allergic flare-ups, I overdid it.

A wonderfully rich cream for very dry and sensitised skin I picked up in Seoul, made of *glycerine*, *ceramides*, *squalane*, *coconut oil* and not much else, was literally the only thing that would not make me break out in itchy welts, so I marinated in it. After about two weeks a lump appeared on my nose that wasn't allergic—it looked and acted more like an impacted pimple. And before I knew it, the suckers were everywhere. My skin still wasn't remotely oily, but I actually managed to develop acne!

I can't complain as the solution was easy. I quit my cream after every skin expert identified *coconut oil* (very nourishing, but exceedingly pore-clogging or comedogenic) as the culprit, and slowly, the pimples disappeared.

But weirdly, I've had to be very careful ever since, having oil-free skincare days regularly so as not to set off any fresh zits (or nodules, as these particular acne lesions are called). It's not logical, given my skin type, but that's skin for you: sometimes it makes no sense.

The moral? Excess of any kind eventually leads to problems. Be kind to your skin. Achieving a balance should be constant aim when looking after it; between water and oil, peeling and slathering, stimulation and fallow periods, deep-cleansing and bacteria—you name it. If you can do that, you're at least halfway there.

BOTTOM LINE: PICK THE LIGHTEST MOISTURISER THAT NONETHELESS KEEPS SKIN HYDRATED ALL DAY

Moisturisers whose ingredients I like:

* Light
Paula's Choice Clear Oil-Free Moisturiser
Clinique Moisture Surge Hydrating Supercharged
        Concentrate
Skinceuticals Metacell Renewal B3

* Medium
Neutrogena Hydro Boost Water Gel Moisturiser
Avène Hydrance UV-Light Hydrating Emulsion
Olay Total Effects Whip Light As Air Moisturiser SPF30
Teoxane Advanced Perfecting Shield SPF30

* Rich
Biossance Squalane + Omega Repair Cream

14 THE SKIN'S LIPID BARRIER / ACID MANTLE / MICROBIOME

YOU NEED TO LOOK AFTER IT

The skin's first line of defence is a slightly acidic veneer made up of skin oils (sebum) and billions of friendly and some less friendly bacteria (the skin microbiome) that thrive in this veneer. It's variously called the lipid or moisture barrier/layer or the acid mantle—same thing, roughly. A colleague compared it to the coating in your non-stick pan.

It naturally locks in moisture and keeps nasty disease- and pimple-causing bacteria out, so it's important. Almost every skin disorder, from acne to eczema to rosacea, is in part the result of a compromised barrier.

In this we are often our own worst enemy. Every

day we rip our skin's barrier apart with aggressive detergents, alcohol, and too many potent anti-ageing ingredients, or scorch it with a lack of moisture. Clever cleansing and intelligent moisturising, however, will stop this daily assault.

And yet sometimes extra daily help may be needed. Pollution, stress, and a rubbish diet are just a few things that can weaken your skin's barrier, while dry and easily-flushed skins often have a genetically less effective one.

In that case, the basic components of the lipid layer are the ingredients to look out for in barrier repair or skin recovery products: *ceramides, cholesterol* and *essential fatty acids*. You'll often find a blend of those.

A few daily drops of *fatty-acid*-rich plant oils such as *rosehip, hemp* or *grapeseed* in your moisturiser can also make your skin less reactive over time. It's a strategy that, a decade ago, took my skin from over-sensitive to normal in the space of a few months of loyal Pai rosehip oil use.

BOTTOM LINE4): A HEALTHY LIPID BARRIER / ACID MANTLE IS KEY IN GOOD SKINCARE

Barrier-restoring products whose ingredients I like:

CeraVe Facial Moisturising Lotion
Curél Moisture Facial Milk
Priori LCA fx140 Barrier Restore Complex

15 STOP PRESS: PROBIOTICS

In medicine, balancing the beneficial microbes that populate our body tissue (some medical researchers estimate that there are 100 trillion of them; they live mainly in our gut) is now seen as a prime new strategy for tackling diseases from IBS to psoriasis or even depression. It is estimated that our body is made up of at least the same number of human cells as non-human cells, if not more of the latter. Yes, it sounds revolting—but these creepy crawlies are keeping you alive and kicking!

Likewise, the microbes that live on our skin are hailed as the latest key to a healthy skin barrier. When it comes to skin we should avoid stripping them with our skincare and instead cultivate the good guys who'll protect us from the bad ones. This is why, increasingly, words such as *probiotic lysate, ferments* and *lactobacillus acidophilus* pop up on INCI lists.

Even if the jury is still out on whether our highly individual bacteria profiles (microbiomes) don't require a more personalised approach for each one of us, this is an interesting field of research in skincare. It certainly looks like probiotic technology in skincare can be a major boon to the health of your lipid barrier.

The prevailing idea is to provide skin with prebiotics, which is food (sugars, fibres) that makes probiotics (friendly bacteria) thrive.

Another strategy is to include fragments of probiotic bacteria, which seem to function as messenger molecules that tell skin cells to behave a certain way.

Products seldom feature actual live bacteria, because it's rather hard to keep them alive, and they stink. What many products do include apart from prebiotics is postbiotics (are you paying attention?).

These are the metabolic by-products (this means, quite literally, poo) of probiotic bacteria that are full of skin-loving actives. Don't worry as they're not microscopic turds; postbiotics take the form of things like lactic acid and ceramides and maintain the protective acidic/lipidic environment of the lipid barrier. It's a bit like the microbes that turn (prebiotic) grape juice into the (postbiotic) by-product that we call wine.

You can find lipid barrier components and probiotics in anything from face mists to moisturis-ers, so you don't necessarily need a specific separate product. Products by brands that specialise in the field of probiotics, such as Gallinée, Mother Dirt and Esse, are the ones I tend to favour.

BOTTOM LINE: PROBIOTICS IS AN UP-AND-COMING AREA OF SKINCARE

Probiotic products whose ingredients I like:
Gallinée Probiotic Hydrating Face Cream
Biossance Squalane + Probiotic Gel Moisturizer
Lancôme Advanced Génifique Sensitive Dual
    Concentrate

16 GOLD STANDARD: SUNSCREEN

THE NO 1 ANTI-AGER

UV is to skin what KFC is to your waistline; there are very few redeeming features. Yes, the sun gives life to many things, keeps depression at bay and we need it to make vitamin D or we'll get brittle bones and limp muscles. As for the latter, roughly 20 minutes' exposure to midday summer sun in the UK three times a week (triple if you have a darker skin as it will deflect more rays) with bare arms and no sunscreen is said to get us enough UV to replenish our vitamin D levels. So there goes that excuse for sunbathing.

Apart from skin cancer, UV's other contributions to your health and your looks are dull skin, age spots, wrinkles, sagging. So incorporating a daily SPF in your routine is standard advice from any skincare expert (who's not French).

It is possibly the best anti-ageing ingredient in the world. It doesn't matter whether you choose a daily moisturiser with an SPF in it, or layer a light SPF lotion over your favourite moisturiser. I have certainly been evangelical about it for the past 20 years.

But SPF is also controversial, and getting more so as time and research go on. For starters, SPF (sun protection factor) only applies to UVB protection. The word has become a shorthand for what in practice should always be 'broad-spectrum UVA/ UVB protection'.

The sunscreen you buy should consist of a minimum SPF30 screen (which protects against UVB induced sun-burn, tanning—a form of DNA damage—and cancer) plus a really good UVA screen (protects against ageing and cancer induced by UVA rays). Look for the word 'broad spectrum protection'. Sometimes it is indicated by a circle with 'UVA' and one to five stars in it. The letters 'PA' followed by one to four pluses, meanwhile, is how sunscreens from Japan, France, and a number of other countries state their level of UV protection.

What you really want is a minimum of four stars or three pluses, especially on the beach (80% of UVA will go through clouds, and it's not reflected by window glass either—up to 75% will reach you if you have a desk near the window). For daily facial sunscreens or moisturisers with sun protection, make sure at least the words 'broad-spectrum' (which guarantees at least the minimum recommended level of UVA protection) and 'SPF30' are involved. Because people use far too little lotion—meaning the SPF level on the bottle is effectively cut in half—the standard SPF15 recommendation for daily use has been cranked up to SPF30 or higher in the past few years.

Of course, if you have darker skin, your skin will have more melanin and therefore more natural protection against UV—some studies say that very dark skin (Fitzpatrick 5/6) has a natural SPF of about 13 (versus an SPF 3 to 4 for Caucasian skin). But that far from means that you're immune from the destruction UV can cause. For starters, your skin is likely to suffer more from uneven pigmentation issues set off or exacerbated by the sun's rays. Never go below SPF20 plus a high UVA rating. Why run the gauntlet if you want to avoid skin damage?

BOTTOM LINE: SUNSCREEN IS THE WORLD'S BEST-ANTI-AGEING INGREDIENT FOR ANY AGE

17 CHOOSING YOUR SUNSCREEN

SOME ARE BETTER THAN OTHERS

Unfortunately, that is not the whole UV story. The two 'physical' sunscreens (meaning they sit on top of the skin, both deflecting and absorbing rays), *zinc oxide* and *titanium dioxide*, are reasonably uncontested and lotions containing these mineral filters are unlikely to irritate your skin.

But they (temporarily) leave a white cast, which is pretty annoying. Also, the darker your skin, the bigger the chance some of this cast will remain visible. If combined with pigmented minerals, these mineral sunscreens do make for great tinted moisturisers or foundations with broad-spectrum protection for light to medium skin, but the choice for darker skins still leaves a lot to be desired.

Chemical sun filters, meanwhile, won't leave a white cast because they sink into skin's top layers, where they absorb UV like melanin does. There are more and more of these, with fetching names like *ethylhexyl methoxcinnamate*—also called, helpfully (not), *octinoxate*—for example.

Their increasing number is a testament perhaps to the search for a chemical sun filter without side effects. It's long been clear that they can irritate sensitive skins, though that's not the biggest issue.

Ironically, some of the longest-used ones like *octrocrylene, oxybenzone* and *avobenzone* can start breaking down in the skin under the influence of UV. The process causes a surge of free radicals, which are rogue atoms that attack healthy cells, resulting in visible damage (ageing) and disease. So that is what is meant when you read (shouty and unhelpful) headlines like, 'Your sunscreen is killing you'.

The breakdown only happens after an hour or two, which is why it is important to reapply sunscreen every two hours when you're in the sun. This should happen anyway, whatever kind of sunscreen you use, because you're likely to rub or sweat a lot of it off over two hours. But in the case of chemical sunscreens, there's this added issue of free radical attack from the inside out. Keep it in mind and just keep re-applying religiously!

If you're not sun-bathing, or when you're outside only sporadically, such as on an office-bound day, your daily face screen should last you the whole day. But the issue has made me think about the daily UV screens I use. Which chemical filters are truly undesirable seems to be a moveable feast (and the newest ingredients have the fewest long-term safety data). For daily use I find myself largely opting for physical filters with pigments instead.

As for the holidays, slapping on any suntan lotion that is available is, hands down, preferable to not using any for fear of smearing 'scary' chemicals on your skin. Unprotected skin will certainly be damaged by that beaming holiday sun. Just make sure the one you use is broad-spectrum, high-factor, and applied over and over generously. I'm talking a third of a 100ml bottle (yes, that much) each time. Just imagine how happy your skin will be not to be blasted to pieces as you are sipping a drink by the pool.

For your face, a dedicated facial SPF will give you less chance of clogged pores. Sunscreens tend to be rich but the industry is working hard at formulas that protect you from UV AND spots. How much should you apply? You should use a (heaped) half teaspoon for your face and neck.

BOTTOM LINE: ANY HIGH-FACTOR SUNSCREEN IS BETTER THAN NO SUNSCREEN

Sunscreens whose ingredients I like:

* Body sunscreens
Superdrug Solait SPF50 Moisturising Sun Lotion
La Roche-Posay Anthelios SPF30 Body Comfort Sun
        Cream
Ultrasun Family SPF30 High Sun Protection

 * Daily facial sunscreens
Avène Tinted Mineral Fluid SPF50
Niod Survival 30 PA+++
Medik8 Advanced Day Total Protect SPF30
Zelens Daily Defence Sunscreen Broad Spectrum SPF30

* Light, oil-free daily facial sunscreens
Dr Sam's Flawless Daily Sunscreen Broad Spectrum
        SPF50
Skinceuticals Ultra Facial Defense SPF50+
PCA Skin Weightless Protection Broad Spectrum SPF45

18 ANTIOXIDANTS

ALWAYS A BONUS

UV and (certain) UV screens aren't the only free-radical fiends. Most foes of your skin set off a demolition party amongst your cells. There's pollution, radiation (blue light from phone and laptop screens, for one), cigarette smoke, alcohol, processed food, the list goes on.

The research on the havoc different types of air pollution (carbon monoxide, nitrogen oxides, particulate matter, and other delights) play with our organs is quite scary. Fortunately, your body makes its own antioxidants (such as *glutathione* and *superoxide dismutase*, which sound like bomb disposal units, which is basically what they are) to neutralise the bastards. A fruit and veg-rich diet brings in much-needed dietary support for your body as a whole. But your skin will get served last and it helps to apply top-ups directly to help the disposal units fighting the free-radicals attacking your dermis. And that's where antioxidant (often abbreviated to AOX) skincare comes in.

Don't get too hung up on which is the most potent antioxidant. There are loads. Most are good, and the key is to use a cocktail of them as different antioxidants tackle different free-radical pathways through which cells get mutated. Ones you will have come across are *green tea, idebenone, vitamins C and E, ferulic acid, Co-Q10*. Any of these are worth including in your daily skincare regime.

They are also an essential part of your sun protection (both the daily and the holiday version), as they hoover up the free radical stragglers that will inevitably break through the UV screen in your suntan lotion. No sun-block can every block 100 per cent of those rays and several lines of defence are needed. Particularly if you live in a city, don't go without them. In any case, start using them from the moment you start wearing daily UV protection (which should be from your teens).

Masses of anti-pollution serums are currently flooding the market claiming to target poisonous particulates in particular. But there is little proof that pitting a special antioxidant against a specific pollutant is effective. Nor is there convincing evidence as yet that blue light requires a specific anti-blue-light antioxidant, as another wave of products will have you believe.

Using a broad-spectrum AOX cocktail is your best bet if you live in an area with pollution in a city. This is one rare example of a type of skincare ingredient where more really is more.

BOTTOM LINE: ANTIOXIDANTS ARE THE FRUIT & VEG OF THE SKINCARE WORLD–INDULGE FREELY

Antioxidant products whose ingredients I like:
The Inkey List Vitamin B, C and E Moisturiser
Paula's Choice Earth Sourced Power Berry Serum
Elizabeth Arden Prevage City Smart
Estée Lauder Advanced Night Repair Synchronised
 Multi-Recovery Complex
Oskia Citylife Concentrate

19 SKINCARE IS LIKE BRUSHING YOUR TEETH

PREVENTION IS BETTER THAN CURE

When I travelled to Korea, I wasn't expecting to be impressed. Patterned obsessively with cartoon designs, everything from the country that made its way to my desk looked like skincare for tweens, and I couldn't get past the cute bears and unicorn colour schemes to study the formulations of the products.

Talking to Koreans, though, I changed my opinion. Good skin to them is holistic: from a health and well-being issue, to a matter of self-respect, rolled into a lifetime project where consistency, gentleness, moisturising and protection are everything. Skin is certainly not something you abuse for years (you always make new skin cells, right?) and then expect to fix with a load of acids, lasers, and miracle ingredients.

And the fact is, Koreans have the secret down pat. It's not very rock 'n roll, but it is very effective. If your skincare is a habit like brushing your teeth, you'll age far more slowly, have fewer instances of psycho skin, and save a fortune on potions and treatments that can only do so much.

Inventors of the double-cleanse and the multi-layered hydration system, the Koreans understand that what we must aim for most of all is protection and prevention. If you'd like people to take you for ten years younger than you are, there is no better way.

BOTTOM LINE: CONSISTENCY AND PROTECTION ARE THE KEYS TO A HEALTHY SKIN

* PART TWO *

PROBLEM-SOLVING ACTIVES

The first part of the book is meant to set you up with a routine that calms your skin, and skincare that doesn't aggravate it but instead nurtures and protects it every day. The products, ingredients and strategies mentioned benefit the health of every skin. They will keep it in good nick if you stick to them for life.

Once you have got your daily regime down to a T, you may feel that there are specific skin issues that you want to tackle. And this is where the world of skincare can become overwhelming pretty swiftly.

As a beauty journalist, I know. Not a month has

gone by in over two decades where I wasn't presented with another 'miracle' formula, innovation or active ingredient. Every so often there was reason for real excitement. But overall few products brought anything truly ground-breaking to the consumer.

This is a world that is so convoluted and preying on hopes and dreams that figuring out each product's merits can be a hard enough task for those whose job it is to keep their finger on the pulse. Separating the wheat from the chaff is particularly tough if the marketing claims are your main focus.

Yet, if you set aside the latest miracle promise, there is a way to figure out what a particular product will undoubtedly do for your skin and this is the focus of this part of the book. You will get to know the problem-solving ingredients that have been proven to work in science and from experience.

These actives are definitely not snake oil. It is the stuff that you can rely on and should look out for when you want to try more than your daily skincare regime.

Stick to these ingredients, with care and attention (that means, choose wisely, don't overdo it and stick to the usage instructions) and you will see results.

There is a caveat. Some of these actives are very potent, meaning the chance of ending up with bouts of sensitivity after using the product increases. It's therefore always best to start from 'mild', treating your skin as delicate and see where that takes you, rather than going nuclear from a standing start to blow your concerns to kingdom come. More likely than not, that approach will throw out the baby with the bathwater.

20 CELL-REGENERATION

PLUMPER SKIN FROM YOUR 30S

Once you hit your 30s, certain 'anti-ageing ingredients' start making sense. Or, as 'anti-ageing' is a dirty word these days, representing a class of products that likes to over-promise and under-deliver, let's call them 'cell-regenerating' ingredients. Your dermis (skin's cell-producing deepest layer) is now getting lazier by the year at producing the *collagen, elastin* and *glycosaminoglycan* (we can call them *GAGs*, phew) cells that form the plump, springy mattress (or 'matrix') of your skin.

The good news is, just as you can prevent middle-age spread by building a bit of exercise into your life, you can keep your skin in shape by training it with the actives that offset the slowdown of the dermis's self-replenishing mechanism.

Problem is, precious few actives can claim to actually affect, let alone penetrate, this deep-lying dermis. And if the ingredient can, there is no guarantee that the serum, cream, mask, mist or whatever potion it's contained in can deliver it.

Whether it can or cannot depends on the concentration of the active ingredient, its delivery system (there are all kinds of elaborate methods to ferry actives deep into the skin, whose foremost job after all is to *keep shit out*), the formula it's contained in, the pH of the product, its packaging, and a ridiculous number of other variables.

This is precisely where the cloak and dagger comes in that's made anti-ageing skincare such a profitable exercise in hopes and dreams—and today, such a target for derision and distrust. So many products have a little of a good active contained in a formula that renders it useless.

Apart from getting a degree in cosmetic chemistry, what can you do?

The answer is to know the (few) actives that do stimulate cell-regeneration, along with the facts what might render them inactive. With that information you'll zero straight in on the limited number of ingredients and products that will keep your skin healthy and great-looking for decades to come.

And hopefully, it'll stop you wasting half your wages on overpriced cold cream in golden jars with crystal spoons.

BOTTOM LINE: CONSIDER CELL-REGENERATION PRODUCTS FROM YOUR 30S

21 'COLLAGEN-BANKING'

STEER CLEAR IN YOUR 20S

An avalanche of (great) new, cheap-ish and disruptive skincare brands has made potent cell-regenerating ingredients more accessible and less mysterious than ever. The direct result is that lots of people are using too many of them too frequently, and too early, and for no good reason. The scourge of the selfie isn't helping: nonstop staring at your face in HD throws up 'imperfections' the naked eye can't see (or that simply aren't there). It also allows for a navel-gazing obsession with egg-like smoothness and carbon-copy facial features if you are of the smartphone generation.

Despite the fact that collagen production technically starts to slacken from your mid-20s, there is no need for anything beyond maintenance and protection for your skin until you get into your 30s (unless you have a skin condition such as *acne* or *rosacea*, more about which in the third part of the book).

Loading up on most of the problem-solving ingredients in this part—such as *peptides, retinol* and high-potency *vitamin C*—before that time is at best a waste of money, and at worst a shortcut to congestion, sensitisation and possibly chronic skin conditions.

So what DO you want to use in your 20s? Well, everything we've discussed in part one, and religiously: consistency, protection and mildness are the keys to having great skin now and for the rest of your life. Humectants, barrier builders, antioxidants, SPF and, if you have spotty skin, salicylic acid, should be in your arsenal from your late teens.

One additional ingredient to look for in your moisturiser or hydrating serum in your twenties, however, is *niacinamide (vitamin B3)*, which appears to be good for anything—it is brightening, barrier-building, pore-refining, soothing and antioxidant. It is also anti-ageing and problem-solving, so you'll find a whole chapter devoted to it in this part of the book.

Others are *panthenol* (*vitamin B5*), which is calming and hydrating. Overall, any inflammatory, calming agents (like *allantoin, azulene, CBD* and *licorice*) are a boon: chronic low-level inflammation is at the heart of all ageing and you're never too young to mitigate it with cell-soothing actives.

BOTTOM LINE: MOISTURE, PROTECTION, AND A GENTLE TOUCH SHOULD BE THE ONLY SKIN STAPLES IN YOUR 20S

Healthy-skin products whose ingredients I like:
YourGoodSkin SPF30 antioxidant Day Cream
CeraVe Facial Moisturising Lotion SPF25
Bioderma Hydrabio Serum Moisturising Concentrate
Medik8 Hydr8 B5 Serum

22 NIACINAMIDE / VITAMIN B3

THE ONE THAT DOES IT ALL

Vitamin B3, or *niacinamide*, is the Renaissance man (sorry, woman) of skincare ingredients. There are no magic bullets in skincare, but this active is close to a magic drop. It can do anything. It helps regulate oil production (bad news for acne and enlarged pores), builds the lipid barrier (minimising irritation, dryness, redness and wrinkles), boosts collagen and elastin production (making it anti-ageing), stops melanin over-production (fading dark spots and even hard-to-tackle melasma or 'pregnancy mask'), and even has some photoprotective (UV-shielding) properties.

You should always be happy to see *niacinamide* on your INCI list. Any concentration will help maintain your skin's health and appearance, but dosages between 2 and 5% have been shown in most of the clinical trials to deliver pleasing results.

It doesn't irritate, penetrates the skin with no problem and is happy to be put in all kinds of ingredient cocktails without throwing its toys out of the pram since it doesn't oxidise (go off) readily, nor does it over-react with other actives. That means it is easy to formulate with. As it is also abundant, a highly effective *niacinamide* formula need not cost much at all (although some brands, of course, will still try to charge you the earth for it).

BOTTOM LINE: LOOK OUT FOR DOSAGES OF NIACINAMIDE BETWEEN 2 AND 5 %

Niacinamide skincare whose ingredients I like:
Garden of Wisdom (GOW) Niacinamide Serum
Dr Sam's Flawless Moisturiser
Olay Luminous Whip Light As Air SPF30 with Niacinamide
Medik8 Clarity Peptides
Paula's Choice 10% Niacinamide Booster

23 PEPTIDES

THE BODY'S SECRET MESSENGERS

Peptides are protein fragments that communicate with cells, signalling to them to start useful processes such as 'make more collagen' and 'stop flaring up'. In the same way that antioxidants neutralise free radicals, there are dozens of cosmetic *peptides* for lots of specific functions that nonetheless work synergistically to do things such as plump out lines and even skin tone. So ideally, you want a cocktail of *peptides*, as opposed to being blinded by the ones that generate the most hype.

Good examples of peptides are Olay's favourite *pentapeptides* (branded as Matrixyl), which can rev up collagen production, and *acetyl hexapeptide-3* (branded as Argireline). The latter is touted to minimise micro-muscle contractions 'just like

Botox', but take that with a bag of salt.

Peptides are non-irritating and have a decent amount of research behind them to prove they are effective at 'correcting' signs of ageing with consistent use. That is as long as they are contained in a formula that manages to help them penetrate deep enough into the skin. Given the substantial size of these molecules, that is anything but straightforward.

So rather than look for creams with a high *peptide* percentage that may do nothing but hydrate the surface of your skin (*peptides* do have great water-binding ability), look for a *peptide* blend along with talk of an advanced delivery system. This is the technology that will actually get the *peptide* mix past the skin's surface.

It could include 'transporter molecules' such as *liposomes*, *smartsomes* or 'cosmetic drones'—no, that's not a joke. Drones are synthetic *peptides* (funnily enough) that have been engineered to carry some actives deeper into the skin and make a pathway for others. They can really supercharge a formula, whether it's based on *peptides* or any other actives that require deep delivery to do their job.

BOTTOM LINE: CHOOSE A PEPTIDE PRODUCT WITH A BLEND OF PEPTIDES AND TALK OF AN 'ADVANCED DELIVERY SYSTEM'

Peptide skincare products whose ingredients I like:
Garden of Wisdom (GOW) Anti-Ageing MultiPeptide
    Serum
Medik8 Liquid Peptides
Drunk Elephant Protini Polypeptide Cream
Niod Copper Amino Acid Serum 2:1
Allies of Skin Peptides & Antioxidants Firming Daily
    Treatment

24 RETINOIDS / VITAMIN A

SKINCARE'S GOLDEN GIRLS

Retinoids are all forms of essential skin vitamin A, which even at low concentrations and in not very active formulas will help skin maintain good health and prevent skin cells from going rogue. Also, the right dose of active vitamin A molecules, of which *retinol* is the most famous, is probably the closest skincare will ever come to an 'elixir of youth'.

Able to rev up the hard-to-reach cells that produce collagen, elastin and other plumping substances, it gets them to behave like pristine, perfectly functioning cells that regenerate more pristine, perfectly functioning cells. Retinoids also prompt surface skin cells to renew in a hurry, pushing plumper, fresher-looking cells to the surface faster. These are processes that happen naturally and plentifully when you're young (that is to say, under 25), but things slowly go south with age and due to environmental damage by the age of 30-35. Over time, use of retinoids will result in improving all the markers of younger, healthier skin: more glow and smoothness, fewer lines, faded dark spots, increased firmness—and also more controlled oil production, smaller-looking pores, and less acne.

So why do we even bother with any other 'anti-agers' or 'cell-regenerators'?

Because in its effectiveness in whipping up improved cell production, *retinol*, the world's most lauded and best-researched cosmetic regenerative ingredient, causes irritation, inflammation, and initial flakiness in a lot of people. Skincare experts will tell you this is only temporary and that you can slowly introduce the vitamin in your regime until your skin gets used to it. That'll be true for many people, but for others the welts and rashes just won't go away. And, as inflammation is massively ageing, they end up with the opposite of a healthy-looking skin.

When I started out as a journalist shortly after the first big wave of cosmetic *retinols*, scientists from all the big skincare companies (Estée Lauder, Clinique, Olay) told me they would 'never go there again.' The side effects of these retinols were so severe (mainly from over-use and not sticking to directions), it was decided that these ingredients were more trouble than they were worth without professional guidance.

Well, more than two decades later, cosmetic *retinols* are once again flooding the market. The good news is that all kinds of advanced buffering and encapsulation technologies have made many retinol formulas more compatible with more people's skins. The bad news is that *retinol* is still a bitch for plenty of others—the less oil-prone you are, the more likely it is that *retinol* will bite.

To mitigate the problem, cosmetic scientists have created many modified *vitamin A* compounds (*retinoids*) over the years, rarely to very impressive effect—until quite recently.

A few newish compounds have been coming

through proper scientific trials with flying colours. It's exciting news for all those people who really want to use a powerful *retinoid* but haven't been able to (like me): we have entered an age where pretty much everyone can benefit from this A* ingredient. So below is an overview of the retinoids that matter.

BOTTOM LINE: RETINOIDS COMBAT EVERY SIGN OF AGEING (AND ACNE), BUT CAN BE IRRITATING TO YOUR SKIN

25 PICKING A RETINOID

Retinoic acid

Also known as *tretinoin* or Retin-A (the brand name), this is the active acid inside *vitamin A* that shocks skin cells into action. It's only available on prescription. If you go to a dermatologist seeking help for acne or advanced sun damage, this is your likely prescription.

It is so potent that at least some redness and flaking is expected for most users. But this ought to subside after a week or two, if you stick to your usage instructions.

It's well-proven that skin can, in many but not all cases, be 'trained' to get used to retinoic acid; so if the medical advice is to use it every third night only at first and to apply only a pea-sized amount, heed it.

If irritation is extreme and persistent, though, immediately go back to your doctor. They might adjust your dosage or put you on a milder *retinoid*. Follow their advice to the letter and don't buy this stuff illegally on the internet!

Retinol

Found in eggs, liver, dairy and plenty of cosmetics, *retinol* converts into *retinoic acid* pretty smartly once applied to the skin (do use a cream and not a slab of meat). This is why its effects (including potential irritation), though a bit slower in manifesting themselves, are so close to those of the pure prescription compound.

But unlike prescription *retinoic acid*, the dosage and formulations of retinol are entirely unregulated. So if you want a *retinol* that actually creates all those magical skin-changing results (these will take two months at least to appear with most skincare actives), you'll have to be a bit of a sleuth.

First of all, make sure it says '*retinol*' not just on the front of the pack but also on the INCI list, and not some word that looks like it, like *retinyl palmitate* (see below), which is a much less potent *retinoid.*

Secondly, dosage is important here. At levels as low as 0.01%, retinol (which is another name for the entire vitamin A molecule) works as a good antioxidant and skin-health preserver, but you won't see wrinkles, bumps and brown spots noticeably diminish. For that, you probably need something ten times stronger, or a minimum of 0.1% retinol—which you can slowly build up to 0.2, to 0.3, to 0.5% (all percentages that are readily available). Without professional guidance, I wouldn't buy anything over 1%. At this strength, your retinol product will show really rapid results but also pose the greatest risk of side effects.

Problem is, most brands don't declare their percentages. This needn't mean their products are lacking in effectiveness, but you might as well go with a product that does tell you how much retinol it contains. Why roll the dice?

But be kind. You're trying to help your skin, not

yank it in a direction. The wise choice is to start low (as in, 0.1% or less) and build up, and pick a sophisticated formula with things like protective *ceramides* and calming agents.

Lastly, retinol is massively unstable and will go off/oxidise/lose its potency if not contained in the right formula and packaging. Try to pick a product in an airless, non-transparent (or dark glass) container. Like all the most potent skincare actives, *retinol* degrades in the presence of light and oxygen. Avoid jars and clear bottles at all costs (this goes for all the *retinoids* in this section, except perhaps *retinyl palmitate*).

Choose one that mentions stability or a stabilising complex; it can be done in a variety of ways but just the mention of stability is a good sign. Slow-release encapsulation will both protect the *retinol* from degrading and prevent an irritating 'spike' of *retinoic acid* hitting your cells.

Retinol products whose ingredients I like:
The Ordinary Retinol (0.5% in squalane)
Beauty Pie Super Retinol Ceramide-Boost anti-Aging

Face Serum (0.09% retinol)
Olay Retinol 24 Night Serum (undisclosed percentage)
Skinsense Retinol Serum (0.3%)
Lancôme Visionnaire Skin Solutions 0.2% Retinol

Retinaldehyde
Retinaldehyde (also called *retinal*) converts into *retinoic acid* even faster than *retinol*, but, oddly, is considerably less irritating.

I can use it, which is saying something as my skin is bothersomely reactive. Scientific evidence also shows that it is biologically more active, turning over cells better than *retinol*. It is also a bacteria killer, making it especially helpful when you have acne.

Retinal's main drawback is that it is impossibly unstable, which is why so few skincare brands are formulating with it. The ones that have done so by using complicated stability complexes, say levels of around 0.05% are the sweet-spot.

Retinal loses its magical powers under the influence of UV. Also, because it's so good at

110

bringing virgin skin cells to the surface, you want to use it only at night and be steadfast about using a minimum SPF30 during the day. The latter is seriously important, and goes for retinoic acid and retinol as much as it goes for retinaldehyde.

Retinal products whose ingredients I like:
Avène Physiolift NIGHT Smoothing Night Balm
Medik8 Crystal Retinal 3
Sarah Chapman Icon Night Smartsome A3X50

Retinyl Retinoate

This Korean-engineered compound is a fusion of *retinoic acid* and *retinol*. As you might expect, it's wonderfully effective (particularly good for improving texture and restoring some firmness) and has the scientific backup (all done on a concentration of 0.06% retinyl retinoate) to prove it.

Inexplicably (well, to me at least) though, it's not at all irritating and, unlike the the retinoids mentioned above, it's stable in UV light, meaning you can use it day and night (although the daytime SPF30+ still applies). The drawback? It's tricky to formulate with and, thus, expensive.

Retinyl retinoate products whose ingredients I like:
Medik8 r-Retinoate Youth Activating Cream
Verso Super Facial Serum

Retinyl Palmitate
If a cream advertises 'vitamin A', it's often this non-irritating, stable compound that needs three steps to turn into *retinoic acid*. It's a good one to have in skincare (even for the under 30s) to keep natural vitamin A in the skin topped up. And, with long-term use, it will help prevent signs of ageing. But claims that it will 'visibly reduce wrinkles in four weeks' (as No7 likes to make for its famous *retinyl palmitate*-based Protect & Perfect serum) is wishful thinking.

In very high doses (Environ Skincare has built its reputation on a 'tiered' system in which you step up our *retinyl palmitate* level over time to consistently normalise cell production) there is a chance of greater improvement, as more of this large molecule may be able to penetrate. But if you're impatient for improvement, your chances of visible results are simply far stronger for the three aforementioned retinoids.

Like some other 'sub-*retinol* retinoids, *retinyl palmitate* is often called a 'pro-retinol', which simply indicates it's a precursor of *retinol* with not quite the same potency or weight of clinical proof behind it.

If you are looking for a potent retinoid that can give speedy results, the word 'pro-retinol' should be a red flag unless it's combined with retinol, as the two might work synergistically.

Retinyl palmitate products whose ingredients I like:
No7 Protect & Perfect Intense Advanced Serum
Environ Skin Essentia Vita-Antioxidant AVST
Moisturiser

A note about bakuchiol
Bakuchiol, an extract from the Indian babchi herb, is not a retinoid. It is not 'natural retinol' in any way and it doesn't function in the same way retinol does. It is however, heavily and misleadingly

marketed and such.

This botanical certainly shows promise: it appears to up-regulate collagen production, making skin smoother, more supple and more even-toned, without causing irritation and flakes. Two (that's not very many) clinical studies have shown these results, based on a concentration of 0.5% bakuchiol.

So: trying any product with 0.5-2% (no less) bakuchiol is not a bad idea at all, in the same way that buying a potent antioxidant is a boon for your skin. Just don't get suckered into thinking you're treating yourself to 'vegan retinol' *eye roll*.

A bakuchiol product whose ingredients I like:
Bybi Bakuchiol Booster

BOTTOM LINE: RETINOIDS ARE DIVA INGREDIENTS THAT REQUIRE CAREFUL CONSIDERATION AND SELECTION

26 ASCORBIC ACID / VITAMIN C

THE ULTIMATE DIVA MOLECULE

Vitamin C is almost as impressive a skincare active as vitamin A, and fraught with almost as many problems.

Like vitamin A, it appears in skincare in a million (okay, about ten) forms, and its effect on your skin is very much dependent not only on the amount of vitamin C, but also the vitamin C compound, and the ingredients it's combined with, and the packaging.

L-ascorbic acid (often abbreviated as '*ascorbic acid*', although the '*l*' guarantees you're dealing with the superior natural, not synthesised, molecule) is to vitamin C what retinoic acid is to vitamin A. It's the active molecule that does all the work. In the case of vitamin C, that work is all about brightening, pigmentation-fading, collagen-synthesising, cell-repairing and free-radical neutralising. And that goes for skin of every colour.

Unlike *retinoic acid, ascorbic acid* is available in skincare without prescription. The problem is, it's maddeningly unstable and starts to oxidise and lose potency almost instantly if any water (aqua on the INCI) is present. Which is a major issue as it's a water-soluble vitamin. It will only be readily absorbed into the skin when delivered in some kind of liquid.

What's more, this preparation has to have a low, acidic pH, or it will neutralise (de-activate) the *ascorbic acid*. That means the potion can be pretty stingy and can make your skin flush. This is, under-standably, interpreted as irritation (it often is not, in fact, but more about that later), and that's never a selling point.

So as with vitamin A, skincare science has come up with a load of alternative vitamin C compounds, both to protect the active molecule from imploding before it gets into the skin and to mitigate the tingling/stinging/burning (delete were appropriate according to your tolerance level/wimpiness).

But compounds like these, with catchy names such as *ascorbyl palmitate, magnesium ascorbyl phosphate, tetra-hexyldecyl ascorbate,* and *sodium ascorbyl phosphate* (I know), generally require conversion after being absorbed in order to release the active goodness. It means the hit of active *ascorbic acid* that actually gets to work on your cells is considerably reduced. And that affects results.

You'll want between 5 and 20% *l-ascorbic acid* and 10% is considered the sweet spot by many experts. If your product has 10% *l-ascorbic acid,* your skin will get all that and you're in clover. However, if the 10% vitamin C advertised on the front of the bottle is actually a compound (that is, you don't see '*l-ascorbic acid*' in the INCI list but something else with '*ascorb*' in it), the dosage you actually get after conversion can be as low as 0.2% *ascorbic acid*—in other words, really very little.

Of the vitamin C compounds, some get considerably more thumbs-up from experts than others. The main tongue-twister to plump for, for being both gentle but with a sustained effect, is *tetra-hexyldecyl ascorbate* (also called, unhelpfully, *ascorbyl tetra-isopalmitate* and, more helpfully, *THD ascorbate*). It is lauded for its ability to penetrate the all-important dermal layer (so it can do its collagen-boosting work) without any irritation. It also appears to have a higher conversion rate than most vitamin C compounds.

Another one, *ascorbyl glucoside*, can be worth a try if combined with specific other actives on the INCI (in particular *niacinamide* / vitamin B3) that boost its effectivity.

Whichever vitamin C compound is used, from the least to the most effective, it will always be marketed as 'vitamin C'. Thankfully all vitamin C compounds are a good thing for your skin and will deliver some protective, brightening and strengthening benefits. In other words, anything on the INCI with *ascorb-* in it can't hurt your chances of healthier skin.

But if you're going to pay big money (say over £30 or $40) in the hope of transforming your skin and expect visible brightening, dark-spot fading and plumping effects in less than a month or two, you'd better make sure you get the high dose of *l-ascorbic acid*.

BOTTOM LINE: TOPICAL VITAMIN C UNDOUBTEDLY IMPROVES SKIN, BUT SOME FORMS AND FORMULATIONS OF VITAMIN C ARE MUCH BETTER THAN OTHERS

27 THE ASCORBIC ACID CONUNDRUM

In practice, by far the best choice for real collagen boosting and visible brightening is pure *l-ascorbic acid* (on the INCI list). So what else do you look for? An airless and opaque pump dispenser is a good start because this active is so perishable. No air or light (which lead to oxidation) must get to the product. Jars are definitely out, no matter how attractive they look or how many little golden spatulas they come with. The key is to look for the formula that's oxidation proof.

Here, there are three options:

Freshly mixed
Some (they used to be rare, but lots have come on the market) formulas are packaged in small vials of

l-ascorbic acid powder that you release into a liquid just before use. As these liquids will contain water to dissolve the ascorbic acid (the lower on the INCI list you spot the word 'aqua', the better), you'll have to use them up over days rather than weeks once you have added the powder.

Some brands have included potent antioxidants and other technologies in the liquid designed to slow the oxidation process down. Either way, when you see the liquid change colour from clear to pale orange and later to brownish orange, you know you've lost the race against time.

You want to stop using it as early as the 'pale orange' stage. A product that is oxidising actually releases damaging free radicals in the skin (much like chemical UV filters after two hours), defeating the point of the product entirely. Skin has some intrinsic ability to turn this process around, but overall, the change in colour indicates that the serum is becoming a pro-ageing one.

As said, you will feel what some euphemistically call 'tingling'. You are applying, after all, a product that is more acid than the pH of your skin. Some might in fact sense a stinging or burning feeling, which can be alarming, especially because we know irritation is bad for skin.

But this is not irritation, it's the skin adjusting to the product's pH, and the feeling should dissipate in a matter of minutes. If a burning sensation does persist or you develop a rash over time, you may have to switch to a less potent option. Or, why not start with a product containing as little as 5% *l-ascorbic acid* and see how your skin responds? In any case, don't let that initial tingle put you off.

Silicone suspension
The powder is 'suspended' (it doesn't quite dissolve and can feel oddly gritty) in a water-free silicone lotion. In itself this isn't the easiest to apply on skin as it doesn't sink in well. But it prevents the powder from being exposed to oxygen and sort of 'attaches' it to the skin so that the *ascorbic acid* can slowly dissolve through its surface, using the water present in the skin.

These suspensions are invariably the stingiest, but

again, any discomfort should subside pretty quickly. Unless you're stupid enough to combine one of these with micro-needling, like I once did on my thighs (don't ask, the life of a journalist is not necessarily a bed of roses). I ended up running around yodelling in agony—it felt like I'd been rolling in stinging nettles. Lesson: a powerful acid plus puncturing small holes in your skin don't mix (obviously).

Ethylated vitamin C
Ethylation (look for '*ethyl ascorbic acid*' in the INCI list) is a process that stabilises *ascorbic acid*, preventing it from degrading even in the presence of water—its greatest foe. No conversion process is needed once an *ethyl ascorbic acid* serum is absorbed into the skin. As with freshly mixed solutions, your cells get the full hit of *ascorbic acid* in the product. This type of solution is very resistant to degradation (you won't see it change colour). It also, in my experience, takes the sting out of the whole process.

Fun fact: pure ascorbic acid stains your hands and nails. The skin on the palms of your hands is harder to penetrate (ditto, obviously, your nails), so some l-ascorbic acid will remain on the surface of the palm or fingers you've applied it to you face with, and oxidise. It means orange/brown hands are proof you've bought a really good vitamin C— but you may want to wash them straight after every application.

BOTTOM LINE: IF YOU'RE GOING TO PAY GOOD MONEY FOR YOUR VITAMIN C, LOOK FOR 'L-ASCORBIC ACID' ON YOUR INCI LIST AND A PERCENTAGE BETWEEN 5 AND 20%

Vitamin C products whose ingredients I like:
Avon Radiance Booster Capsules (20% l-ascorbic silicone suspension)
The Ordinary Ethylated Ascorbic Acid (15% solution)
Tandem Brightening Booster (THD ascorbate 20%)
Murad Vita-C Eyes Dark Circle Corrector (l-ascorbic acid and THD ascorbate)
Clinique Fresh Pressed Daily Booster with Pure Vitamin C (10% l-ascorbic acid)
Alumier MD Ever Active C&E+ Peptides (15% l-ascorbic acid)

28 EXFOLIATING ACIDS

BOTH ACE AND A MINEFIELD

The problem with acids is that they work, quickly and noticeably. Which gets people over-excited and happy to over-use them, which leads to irritation and dryness.

Like retinol, cosmetic acids first enjoyed great popularity some 20 years ago, but were discontinued the by big brands as consumers went way overboard with them. Today's 'new wave' of acids is more sophisticated and in many cases better formulated, but the results-hungry public is still more than capable of over-doing them.

Use acids properly and they will dissolve the 'glue' that allows dead skin cells to outstay their welcome, a process that helps hydrate, fades pigmentation and dullness, and stimulates collagen production.

The first things you will see are less dull, glowier skin and possibly fewer spots, which explains why people immediately want to bathe in the stuff.

When you hear people banging on about using acids on their face, they are referring to exfoliating or cell turnover-boosting *alpha, beta* and *polyhydroxy acids (AHA, BHA* and *PHAs)*.

There are legion, all doing a similar job but all with a slightly different USP, so on the whole it's a far better idea to select a product with a great blend of acids than one with an impressive-sounding percentage of just one.

Some (but not all) of them are:

Salicylic acid: the only *BHA*, this birch tree extract (now mostly synthesised), is fat-soluble which allows it not only to peel the skin surface but to get into and unplug pores. It's also anti-inflammatory and antibacterial, making it both one of the gentlest acids and the most effective when it comes to spots and congestion.

Lactic acid: derived from milk, it has great affinity with skin as our bodies make *lactic acid*, as do the good bacteria that populate our skin in their billions. It is potent, but generally great for sensitive skin if you don't overdo the dosage.

Azelaic acid: not an AHA, BHA, or PHA, it still works as a leave-on exfoliant that can smooth rough texture and lines. But importantly, it's so effective as an antibacterial and anti-inflammatory that it's become a favourite for treating acne and rosacea. It also slows down the formation of melanin so it's great for treating hyperpigmentation.

Mandelic acid: a gentle exfoliator and pore-clearer with antibacterial properties. Compared to its pore-clearing brethren *azelaic* and *salicylic acid*, it carries the lowest risk of lightening skin or causing irritation resulting in post-inflammatory hyperpigmentation, so it's a good choice for spot-prone, dark skin tones.

Malic acid: a peeling agent that boosts *ceramide* production (helping to strengthen the protective lipid layer) and inhibits melanin production, reducing dark spots.

Citric acid: can be irritating as an exfoliator and brightener but also acts as a chelator, meaning that it nukes environmental irritants such as heavy metals and other pollutants, so is a good choice for city dwellers.

Phytic acid: a gentle, slow-release acid that's effective against pigmentation and particularly good at unclogging pores and dealing with blackheads. It's also a chelator.

Polyhydroxy acids: these are so-called 'second and third-generation acids' (the first generation being *AHA's/BHA*), and you'll find them listed as *lactobionic acid, gluconolactone* and *maltobionic acid.* Their action, thanks to their slightly larger molecule size that penetrates slowly but surely— is so gentle, there is no chance of irritation even if used every day.

Yet they're highly effective at increasing cell turnover and hydration, thanks to their added ability to attract and hold water.

Other boons include antioxidant protection, chelating action, dark spot-slaying, and an ability to protect cells from UV damage as well as glycation (stiffened, malformed protein fibres, read 'wrinkles', thanks to sugar consumption). Of all the *acids, polyhydroxies* are the least likely to cause problems, even if you have sensitive skin and/or you use them every day in multiple products.

Glycolic acid: derived from sugar, it's the smallest acid molecule, allowing it to sink deeper and faster into the skin than others and showing the most visibly line-reducing and overall quickest results. No wonder every skincare brand feels it must offer some kind of glycolic 'wonder' product.

Unfortunately, the molecule is so small it's capable of worming its way between not only dead cells but healthy cells as well, making it the most prone to causing irritation and inflammation. One dermatologist I know calls it the 'sledgehammer of acids'. She, as do others, avoids using it as there are plenty of other acids without this drawback.

Don't use it indiscriminately and if you know your skin is sensitive, avoid it. If you have dark skin and are prone to hyperpigmentation, proceed with caution.

BOTTOM LINE: GLYCOLIC IS THE FASTEST-ACTING AND MOST AGGRESSIVE COSMETIC ACID; POLYHYDROXIES ARE THE MILDEST

29 HOW TO USE ACIDS

So how do you take your acids? Well, any which way, it seems, as they now lurk in almost every type of product, making overdoing it all too easy if you don't pay attention.

So don't follow an acid toner with an acid serum, for example, or an acid cleanser with an overnight acid mask. The exception to this rule is a salicylic acid cleanser and toner combo, which is beneficial for spotty skin.

For most people, applying an exfoliating acid three times a week, however, is plenty, in the same way that you wouldn't use a scrub every day. Yes, there are some who swear by using an acid toner daily. It's certainly beneficial if skin needs extra help shedding dead cells, for example if it's oily and congested or ageing and therefore slow in turning over.

But people with normal, dry and sensitive skin (I speak from experience) should go for a less-is-more approach or their skin will flare up eventually. As you'll know by now, I believe your starting point should always be to treat your skin as delicate in the first instance.

The skin cells of anyone under 30 without any discernible congestion of their skin, meanwhile, do plenty of turning over by themselves. There is simply no need for sustained peeling as at best you're wasting your money, and at worst you're setting yourself up for problems in the future, including not only sensitisation but sun damage as well.

That's because constant exfoliation means you MUST keep your face out of the sun altogether, which few people manage to do. Over-aciding combined with UV radiation is a sure-fire route to uneven pigmentation and wrinkles.

Polyhydroxy acids (PHAs) are the one exception, as they boost cell turnover without sensitising skin or making it vulnerable to sun damage, and have hydrating and protective properties any skin can benefit from.

Aciding options are:

Acid cleansers
How intense a peel these provide depends not only on the types and levels of acid, but also on how long it's left on the skin. Massaging in a cleansing balm featuring acids will give you more of a hit than using a wash-off cleansing foam. Either way, this is a relatively low-impact way to incorporate acids. Just be sure not to use this on your eyes.

Acid cleansers whose ingredients I like:
Salicylic acid: CeraVe SA Smoothing Cleanser
Salicylic, glycolic acid: Murad AHA/BHA Exfoliating
Cleanser
Glycolic, phytic acid: Dennis Gross Alpha Beta Pore
Perfecting Cleansing Gel

Acid toners
Don't get these mixed up with regular toners, even if those sometimes use a low level of lactic acid to re-balance your skin's pH. When a toner or lotion

specifically markets itself as an 'acid' or 'anti-pig-mentation' or sometimes 'brightening' tonic, listing its acids boldly, you're dealing with a liquid peel that can be quite potent as it sinks in instantly and stays on your skin.

Acid toners whose ingredients I like:
Salicylic acid: Paula's Choice 2% Salicylic Acid Toner
Lactic acid: REN Ready Steady Glow Daily AHA Tonic
Lactic, phytic acid: Sarah Chapman Skinesis Liquid
        Facial Resurfacer

Acid peeling pads
These are acid toners in pad form, often incorporating a blend of acids. As with toners, don't wander out without SPF after using them and consider limiting their use to two or three times weekly if they're AHA-based and even if they're marketed for daily use. Some employ a two-step system, first the application of a high level of grime and dead cell-dissolving acids, followed three minutes later by a pad impregnated with neutralising solution to stop the acid over-doing things. This is all very delicately worked out by your acid pad purveyor, so make sure you stick to the exact timings as written in the usage

instructions. This two-step system is how professional peels work, so they are a clever buy. But you should definitely see them more like a peel or mask, and not make them a daily habit without professional supervision.

Acid pads whose ingredients I like:
Lactic acid, PHA: Alex Steinherr x Primark Pollution
     Solution Dual Texture Exfoliating Pads–60 pads
Salicylic, lactic, malic acid: Dr Dennis Gross Alpha Beta
     Universal Daily Peel–5 pads
Salicylic acid: Aveda Outer Peace Acne Relief Pads–50
     pads

Acid serums
Deeply absorbed and often with (much) higher acid percentages than toners, these can certainly leave your skin flushed—but also more even-toned. Primarily used overnight as they make you very sun-sensitive, they shouldn't be used on a daily basis (even if you keep reading breathless statements from your peers who do so—it won't be long before they change their minds). PHA serums are the exception, as they don't make the skin more susceptible to sunburn.

Acid serums whose ingredients I like:
Garden of Wisdom PHA+ serum
Oskia Liquid Mask Lactic Acid Micro-Peel
Allies of Skin Mandelic Pigmentation Corrector Night
    Serum

Acid moisturisers

Wearing a cream with AHA's (*glycolic, malic* etc.) as a daily moisturiser carries a risk of sensitisation and sun damage, even if you're good about your sunscreen—which must be why acid moisturisers are *really* hard to find in the UK (there are plenty of them in the US, if you are desperate, which I wouldn't be). *AHA* night creams are thin on the ground as well; if you want to use one, commit to reapplying plenty of SPF50 throughout the day. A PHA (*lactobionic, gluconolactone*) hydrator is safe, though.

Acid moisturisers whose ingredients I like:
Salicylic acid: La Roche-Posay Effaclar Duo Moisturiser
PHA: Neostrata Restore Bionic Face Cream
Glycolic, lactic, salicylic acid: Glamglow Good In Bed
    Passionfruit Softening Night Cream

Acid masks

These are not supposed to be left on longer than 20 minutes or used more than once a week. So, despite often employing some of the highest levels of acids, they cause few issues and can be a real pre-big-day or pre-party perker-upper. But have a trial run first to make sure to see how your skin reacts.

Acid masks whose ingredients I like:

Salicylic, glycolic, lactic acid: Beauty Pie Super Pore Detox Black Clay Mask

Lactic, mandelic acid: Environ Tri Biobotanical Revival Masque

Lactobionic acid: Zelens Transformer Instant Renewal Mask

BOTTOM LINE: IT'S EASY TO OVERDO ACIDS, SO DON'T GO MAD OR YOU'LL SENSITISE YOUR SKIN

30 ACID PERCENTAGES ARE MISLEADING

Like those chilli-eating contests where people show off who can consume the hottest pepper without their head exploding, acid level one-upmanship has become sort of a badge of honour for brands. It's the kind of clamour that could make you feel there's something wrong with you if you're an anything-less-than-10%-*glycolic* kind of woman. While there are areas where percentages of the active ingredient can be discriminating guides, this isn't one of them.

On the one hand a she-woman approach to exfoliation can lead to angry-skin issues, and on the other hand these numbers can distort what the product really does.

One thing that sometimes happens is that a brand

will state eye-catching percentages of acids but will pack their product full of buffering or neutralising agents (examples are *sodium bicarbonate, sodium lactate, potassium hydroxide, sodium phosphate, triethalonamine* and *glycine*). These are always present in acid products to stabilise the pH of the formula— which is a good thing, as the pH controls the potency and penetration of the acid. But at high levels they mean that some or even most of the acid, though present, is neutralised before it gets to your skin. You think you are buying a strong peel, but, instead you are getting a mild exfoliator.

While satisfying the consumer's appetite for a potent-looking percentage, brands this way simultaneously sidestep mass irritation (what is bad for skin is also bad for business). It also means formulations stay on the right side of the very strict EU regulations that govern the safety of cosmetic formulas. While the amount of acid is correct, the pH and the neutralising agents present ensure the product is much less intense, and therefore safer, than you might have bargained for. So you can see the smoke and mirrors going on here. It's certainly not what all brands do. But it happens.

Figuring all this out from your INCI list requires, frankly, a cosmetic chemistry degree. Having said that, one handy hack if you're going to pay for a potent peel is to make sure you spot the acids you are after near the top of the list and your buffering agents near the bottom, or in a separate 'neutralising' solution, as with professional and some at-home peels.

Much better, though, is not to make some number on the front of the bottle your guiding principle when choosing an exfoliator. What drives your choice should be the type of product you are looking for. Are you looking for a daily toner or a weekly mask? The other determining factor should be the result you are hoping to achieve with the acid or acid blend that's right for your skin: *salicylic* to combat oiliness or a blend of *PHA*'s to hydrate and brighten?

It should be led by whether you trust the brand. An established skincare brand will create a formula of many ingredients besides the acids, such as calming agents and barrier-builders, that will optimise the acid *and* the overall health of your skin.

And you should be willing to experiment, to a degree. Start slowly, and you will soon learn whether that's all your skin needs or if it thrives on a more thorough approach.

You should always stick rigidly to the usage instructions (exactly how much product, how often, how long for). They are there for a reason when you're playing with potent cosmetic actives! Gung-ho use of acids will weaken and upset skin. But correct use will make it stronger and healthier over time.

BOTTOM LINE: PRIORITISE THE RIGHT TYPE OF ACIDS FOR YOUR SKIN, NOT THE ACID PERCENTAGE ON THE BOTTLE

* PART THREE *

ISSUES

This part deals with particular issues and trends that I am always asked about. This includes the right order for the dazzling array of products that are available, how to make sure you invest your hard-earned cash in a great product, and how superior 'natural' cosmetics really are (or not). You'll also find strategies here for tackling really annoying and upsetting skin issues such as acne, rosacea and psoriasis.

31 UNEVEN PIGMENTATION

There are several reasons for your skin tone becoming uneven and acquiring brown spots, or 'pigmented lesions'. One is hormonal pigmentation, caused by, among other things, pregnancy, or the Pill. The result often is melasma, or 'pregnancy mask': large pigmented areas that are quite deep and quite hard to treat (but that can also suddenly disappear).

Another one is post-inflammatory hyperpigmentation, where inflammation or trauma to the skin causes a surge of melanin with a resulting dark blotch. Darker skins are particularly vulnerable to this, especially those suffering from acne, which comes with lots of inflammation (so, taking a calming, anti-inflammatory rather than an aggressive approach to spots, and refraining from picking at your skin at all costs, is even more important for those with darker skin than it is for everyone else).

But the number one cause of discolouration is UV exposure. Most of your brown spots have been multiplying and lying in wait under the surface of your skin since you first stepped into the sun unprotected. Once you reach your 30s (or sometimes a lot sooner, if you've really been caning it sunbathing-wise), they will come out of hiding. The best thing to stop them from multiplying, at any age, is a daily sunscreen and additional care when you are on a holiday in the sun.

When I grew up, this kind of discolouration was seen as a mark of enjoying a good life with a 'healthy' dose of sunbathing, or simply as freckles (which are an entirely different thing, unrelated to damage or advancing years).

As a budding journalist, I wrote about wrinkles and skin that sagged, but hardly ever about brown spots. Then, quite suddenly, the big skincare brands started to talk pigmentation to us beauty journalists. Research had shown, they told us, that the human eye perceives skin with blotches as more aged, even, than a skin covered in lines and wrinkles.

Help, obviously, was at hand, in the form of the miracle potions the brands had formulated to tackle the problem, borrowing heavily from the South-East Asian Market, where the reverence of porcelain skin had long since produced countless skin-whitening and brightening strategies. To this day, I marvel at how successfully and how quickly this message whipped us, and consequently the consumer, into a frenzy over pigmentation. Within months it was a thing, and today, everyone seems to be aware of every single blotch and dark spot.

The truth is that once a brown spot has become visible on your skin, it's a pain to fade with mild cosmetics. Aggressive lightening ingredients such as hydroquinone (available in cosmetics in the US but on prescription only in Europe) may, thanks to the risk of irritation, do more harm than good in the long run, especially when unsupervised by a physician. Elsewhere, people have been disfigured by horrible unregulated or illegal skin bleaches.

The way forward, it seems, is a mix of powerful ingredients that either hamper the formation of melanin (called tyrosinase inhibitors; examples are *licorice, arbutin, b-resorcinol* and *tranexamic acid*) or break up the existing pigment (*vitamin c, retinol, azelaic acid, AHA's, niacinamide*). These come in multiple permutations from a selection of different brands, many of them looking pretty effective, potentially, if you commit to using them consistently.

I have to be honest, though. You almost always need to combine such lightening cosmetics with some form of clinical treatment such as lasers or professional peels to significantly reduce brown spots. For melasma, oral *tranexemic acid* tablets show a lot of promise, but you'll need to consult a dermatologist for guidance and a prescription.

And if you don't cover your skin at the same time with an SPF30 to 50 every single day, you might as well flush your money down the toilet.

If you're in your 20s or younger, you are in luck.

There's only one thing you need to do to not get brown spots at a later age: use a good sunscreen daily (and don't sunbathe). Think you're immune? Just you wait!

BOTTOM LINE: WITHOUT SUN PROTECTION, TREATING HYPERPIGMENTATION IS POINTLESS

Promising pigment faders whose ingredients I like:

Neostrata Enlighten Illuminating Serum (licorice, niacinamide)

SkinCeuticals Discolouration Defense Serum (tranexamic acid, kojic acid)

Allies of Skin Mandelic Pigmentation Corrector Night Serum (AHA, niacinamide)

Elequra Radiance Accelerator Serum (retinol and vitamin C)

32 REDNESS IS A TREND

Judging from my in-crate, the whole world is now suffering from some level of skin irritation or redness or even the skin disorders rosacea, eczema, and psoriasis. Although there is no definitive explanation, the usual suspects are pretty self-evident. There's genetics (dry, thin, Celtic skins are first in line for problems, but everyone else's is next).

Another reason is over-enthusiastic use of aggressive or age-inappropriate products and treatments such as *acids* and *retinols*, and even professional peels and lasers. And then there is stress and, in the cities, rampant pollution. Both set off a cascade of events in the skin that can lead to chronic redness. So does a lack of sleep, a poor diet, and a work-hard-play-hard lifestyle. Oh, and the psychological pressure of having to keep up with the Insta-Joneses, combined with, increasingly, a lack of stress-relieving physical contact with real friends, is not helping at all. These are the realities of life we're hardly going to overcome anytime soon, so it pays to know how to either prevent or quell a flaring face.

First, let's distinguish between sensitised (or reactive) skin, which you can tackle yourself, and skin disorders such as eczema and psoriasis, which can't really be cured but can get worse over time if they're not managed with some professional support.

If you suffer from itchy, warm, red (if you have dark skin, the colour is more violet, if it's visible at all), rashes on a regular basis—ones that appear on different areas of your face without a discernible reason—your skin is probably sensitised.

This means its protective lipid barrier has become compromised, and that the products and ingredients that your skin was once absolutely fine with are suddenly setting off sirens in your cells.

Anything can start the process, but the most likely culprits are often known irritants such as fragrance, alcohol, acids, and certain preservatives, emulsifiers and detergents.

My first sensitised-skin episode was when I suddenly started suffering from bright red, weeping armpits as I was working night-TV shifts on my first job. My sleeping pattern stressed my body and weakened its defences. I bought a new deodorant with a 'gentle' fragrance, which was a pointless exercise. It took quite a few weeks before I got that my skin was no longer going to put up with fragrance of any kind.

Over the years, both my facial and body skin have treated me to furious reactions to all kinds of ingredients, always out of the blue, but usually in times of some type of stress.

As I learned to re-enforce my lipid barrier-slash-acid mantle and never to undermine it with all the stuff that does, my skin has got far more resilient, which means I can now use some active ingredients, such as retinoids, that an acutely sensitised skin cannot cope with. But getting to that point meant respecting my skin and getting to know very well what ingredients to look for and which ones to avoid.

If your redness tends to be like a warm, red (or purplish) flush in a sort of 'butterfly' shape across your cheeks, T-zone and chin, you may have rosacea and you need to work even harder at managing it. If you don't, it can get worse; the redness could deepen into permanently dilated veins, and you could also develop lumps and acne-like lesions which are really upsetting and hard to treat.

Nobody really understands what causes rosacea (genes, certain bacteria and skin mites, and neurovascular irregularities may have something to do with it). Like acne, if it worries you it deserves some pro attention at an early stage, so you can control it under the supervision of a medical expert.

The same goes for eczema (raw, weeping, relentlessly itchy scabby patches 'thanks' to an overreacting immune response) and psoriasis (an auto-immune disorder with potential allergic and genetic triggers that makes skin over-produce cells, creating thickened, scaly, moist patches). Both need a doctor's attention and prescription medication alongside the same calming and healing approach to skincare you should apply to flaring, angry skin of any kind.

BOTTOM LINE: TO FIGHT ANY TYPE OF IRRITATION OR SENSITISATION, YOU NEED TO TREAT SKIN WITH RESPECT FOR LIFE, NOT JUST FOR CHRISTMAS

33 HOW TO BEAT SAID TREND

Frankly, you already know how to go about calming skin: the rules for ultra-gentle cleansing, respectful moisturising, and barrier-building apply. Doing so can make sensitised skin act normal again and keep rosacea from getting worse, but it has to be a life-long commitment rather than a sticking-plaster few weeks of doing the right thing! Chuck out anything (including makeup!) with sulphates, alcohol, fragrance, 'cooling, calming' essential oils (they in fact have the opposite effect) such as mint and menthol, along with face scrubs and cleansing brushes. All of these will aggravate your lipid barrier, and that is the root of your problem. Any sulphate-free cleanser (used with tepid water—hot water strips skin of lipids) suited to your skin type is the right choice. But if your delicate skin is dry (as is often the case), you may be a good candidate for a fragrance-free cleansing oil. If it's plant oil-based, it will have the added benefit of supplying some essential fatty acids (plant oils particularly high in these are *sea buckthorn, rosehip, squalane, chia*) which are important for helping re-construct a barrier that's sprung holes. Other great barrier-enforcing ingredients (as they are natural con-stituents of a healthy barrier) are ceramides, cholesterol and pre- and probiotics, along with glycerin, which both attracts water to the skin and keeps it from evaporating. It used to be a bit of a slog to find a blend (a mixture is better than a single one) of these in a moisturiser. But with the rocketing increase of flaring skin, barrier-repair cleansers and serums are part of many a brand's skincare offering. Meanwhile, ranges specifically geared towards dry, sensitive skin will often have these ingredients as standard (although, remember—if they also feature *alcohol, sulphates* or *fragrance*, your skin is not going to like you). They may also include active calming ingredients, proven to take down redness and mitigate inflammation. Often derived from botanicals known for being soothing, like camomile and oats, words to look for are *allantoin, beta-glucan, bisabolol, azulene, colloidal oatmeal, licorice, curcumin, CBD, panthenol* and *green tea.*

Because already-sensitised skin really can't take the added onslaught of UV, it is especially important for your skin that you wear an SPF30 at least (whatever your skin colour). Choose a mineral (or physical) formula, featuring zinc oxide and/or titanium dioxide, to minimise any chance of further irritation and make sure it's fragrance-free as well. This may take some careful INCI scrutiny of products as 'natural' mineral formulas tend to be keen on throwing in essential oils, which are a bastard for sensitised skin.

BOTTOM LINE: BARRIER-BUILDING AND INFLAMMATION-CALMING PRODUCTS FOR IRRITATED SKIN ARE EASY TO GET BY THESE DAYS

34 TYPES OF REDNESS

TARGETED HELP

There are things you can do beyond your core calming regimen. In that case it will help if you understand your specific inflammatory condition better.

Sensitivity
Rashes that keep appearing for no obvious reason probably mean you've developed a sensitivity to a specific ingredient, which you'll have to root out. Unfortunately, the irritant could be anything under the sun (some people become sensitive to water) so try to strip back your regime to the most basic (meaning no *colour, fragrance*, or active ingredients at all) cleanser and moisturiser—CeraVe, Curél and La Roche Posay Toleriane are some good ranges for sourcing these.

Then re-introduce actives one by one to see which your skin protests against (this is where an INCI 'skin diary' in which you keep track of all ingredients in your products seriously helps; that's how I figured out that coconut oil was giving me nodules).

Apart from all the sensitisers already mentioned in this chapter, *chemical sunscreens, lanolin* (if you have a wool allergy), *PEG* and *PPG* (petrochemical emulsifiers) and *MI* or *MIT* (an alternative preservative that has turned out to be far more irritating than the much, and often unjustly, maligned parabens) are a few things to keep an eagle eye out for, as they are known to cheese many skins off.

If your flare-up is particularly bothersome and you can't wait days for it to calm down, the failsafe way to settle it is 1% hydrocortisone, which you can get over the counter at the pharmacist. Hydrocortisone can thin the skin, among other side effects, but this is only the case if you use lots of it for days or weeks on end. For acute inflammation due to a reaction to some irritant, a tiny dab of hydrocortisone once or twice in 24 hours won't hurt you, and it will make your rash vanish in the space of hours. Just keep a tube for emergencies and treat it as such.

Rosacea

If you suspect your insistent, warm-feeling redness is rosacea, get on the case immediately, as treating it from the onset can stop its progression (flushing developing into permanently dilated veins, bumpy or flaky skin) and makes it much easier to control.

Surprisingly, there are two acids that, far from aggravating the condition, have been shown to help it: a daily serum or lotion with 2% *salicylic* or 10% *azelaic* (the highest amount you can get in a cosmetic) can settle redness and flakes.

Vitamin C is important for strengthening skin and warding off inflammation, but be careful with the really potent *l-ascorbic* acid formulations. If they sting, they can make matters worse. A non-stingy but effective vitamin C compound such as *THD ascorbate* would be a good starting point.

But avoid other potent products, such as *AHA peels*, high-strength *retinol* serums and *hydrocortisone* which can aggravate the situation.

If things don't settle or you develop *acne rosacea*, where pimples are added to the equation, you should seek medical attention. A dermatologist will likely put you on prescription meds (prescription-strength 15% *azelaic acid*, a low-dose *retinoid*, and *antibiotic gel* are options) that could help.

You could could consider a course of IPL (Intense Pulsed Light) or vascular laser to make veins collapse, diffusing the redness in the upper skin layers. It works, but it's expensive and not permanent.

Super-gentle yellow, red and near-infrared LED light therapy (using specific wavelengths that, unlike UV light, have benefits without DNA-destroying drawbacks), meanwhile, can really calm redness and heal aggravated skin, if you have regular sessions.

This is one of the few instances where investing in an at-home device can pay dividends. Unlike most gadgets, which in my experience get used for two weeks before ending up in the back of the cupboard with the ice cream maker, the best LED masks are such a joy and simple to use, you'll actually stick to getting your daily few minutes of healing light.

Soothing products for sensitive and rosacea-prone skin I like:
CeraVe Hydrating Cleanser
La Roche-Posay Toleriane Sensitive Crème
Garden of Wisdom (GOW) Neurophroline Serum
Niod Survival 30 PA+++ Silicone-Dispersed UV Minerals
Pai Instant Calm Chamomile & Rosehip Calming Day Cream
SkinCeuticals Redness Neutralizer
iS Clinical Pro Heal Serum Advance Plus
Dr Dennis Gross DRx Spectralite FaceWare Pro LED Mask

Eczema

Eczema can be much helped with a core calming regime. Apart from everything already discussed, avoid *parabens* and *MI* preservatives and cut out *AHA*'s and any *retinols* as well, as they'll just cause more upset around eczematic lesions.

But eczema will still rear its ugly head randomly whenever it fancies. Because it leaves skin open and desperately vulnerable, it needs seriously skin-sealing, protective moisturisation. This is where, traditionally, mineral oil/soft paraffin/petroleum jelly has come into its own. Yes, it is a so-called petrochemical, but its cosmetic-grade version is purified, not toxic, and completely inert, which means it's not doing anything but forming a clingfilm-like occlusive layer over the skin, keeping much needed water and lipids in the skin. It's the basic component of all those creams in the 'eczema isle', such as E45 and Diprobase.

There is another school of thought, however, that says that any petrochemical derivatives can worsen the discomfort and itching that conditions like eczema and psoriasis bring, so they should be avoided in favour of (fragrance-free) creams based on rich plant butters such as *shea, cocoa* and *mango*.

So who's right? The camps are diametrically opposed. I use cosmetic-grade mineral oil-based creams to beat back eczema patches on my body (on the face, both mineral oil and rich plant oils can cause congestion and need to be used cautiously) and find them very useful. But I first layer an *unscented, fatty acid*-rich oil such as *squalane* under them so the former can nourish and help heal while the latter keeps things from getting worse. Alternatively, I use creams that combine some *mineral oil* with *fatty acid*-rich oils, *glycerine, ceramides* and/or anti-inflammatories such as *colloidal oatmeal* to get the best of all worlds.

If the problem persists or gets worse, the doctor may prescribe a short course of a prescription *corticosteroid* (such as *hydrocortisone*). Always use only ever for as long as directed on the prescription, and not longer (don't self-medicate). It can stop the vicious circle of inflammation, weeping and scabbing and give skin a chance to heal, which is a damn sight better than just letting the condition rage and weaken your skin.

Apart from the right *corticosteroid*, a doctor could prescribe phototherapy, which involves controlled exposure to UVA or UVB light, sometimes combined with medication. UV light can help reduce eczema symptoms, but for obvious reasons (ie, UV light seriously damages skin's DNA), this is only suitable for pretty bad and chronic eczema cases.

Eczema soothers for the body whose ingredients I like:
Aveeno Skin Relief Nourishing Lotion with Shea Butter
Cetraben Natural Oatmeal Cream
La Roche-Posay Lipikar Baume AP+
CeraVe Moisturising Cream

Psoriasis
Under the scaly layers of skin that psoriasis brings, there is inflammation and irritation, so you need to carefully balance the absolute need to calm the situation while trying to slough off the dead cells. *Salicylic acid*, thanks to its anti-inflam-

matory powers, is very well suited to this, so it's worth trying a daily 2% *salicylic acid* gel on the affected area and see how you go.

A good *retinoid*, meanwhile, normalises skin function, mitigating the excessive cell growth. But you'll have to experiment to see how sensitive your skin is to it; if it irritates yours, it will cause more harm than good. You should start on a low-dose *retinol* or a gentle alternative like *retinyl retinoate* and build up from there.

Alternatively, you may want to stick *fatty acid*-rich lipids and anti-inflammatories to soothe the skin as much as possible, but that won't get rid of the scaliness.

And don't forget a daytime mineral SPF30 on any exposed skin including your lesions (this goes for psoriasis as well as eczema); you don't want this damaged skin to suffer further UV attack.

Overall, psoriasis is a nasty skin disease that needs careful managing, with a dermatologist to help oversee this if the problem persists.

Corticosteroids are a medical option here as well (although you want to go easy), as are vitamin D-based medications (a lack of vitamin D is common in people with chronic psoriasis) and the UV and LED light therapies mentioned previously.

BOTTOM LINE: DIFFERENT INFLAMMATORY SKIN CONDITIONS NEED DIFFERENT TREATMENT: IF IN DOUBT, SEE A DOCTOR

35 ACNE

THERE IS NO CURE YET (SORRY)

We can untangle the human genome and put a man on the moon, but we don't exactly understand why acne happens, and we can't cure it. It's a rubbish state of affairs, especially when it looks like we're in the midst of an acne epidemic. That's according to every dermatologist I know. They all report significantly increased rates of people in all age brackets seeking help. Official estimates vary, but it's thought globally over 80% of people under 30 suffer from breakouts, while a conservative estimate (others point to much higher figures) says that 25% of women over thirty is affected by some level of acne.

Despite the issue not being fully understood, the contributing factors are well-known, and that's where we can learn to control the thing, even if not fully make it go away.

Hormones are clearly a central issue. Any fluctuation throwing their balance out of whack, and causing a sudden spike in androgens (male hormones), will make skin produce more oil. And that can lead to blocked pores and spots. This explains why there are more women suffering from adult acne than men; our hormones fluctuate far more wildly throughout life than men's.

Any medications that increase androgens such as testosterone are an acne trigger as well. As are your genes (thanks, mum and/or dad) and hormone-disrupting realities of modern life such as poor sleep, stress and food full of hormones.

About as bad as hormones is inflammation—and this is something we really can tackle. Anything that irritates or inflames the skin or the gut is going to make acne worse, because acne is primarily an inflammatory disorder.

And there is one particular lifestyle cause that's not

often mentioned but that experts point to as a huge reason for persistent spotty breakouts around the hairline, jaw and neck: styling products. That's hairstyling products, replete with waxes, synthetic oils and silicones that will seep into the hairline and sweep over the sides of congestion-prone faces. Over time, regular breakouts can turn into persistent acne if not tackled, so it's worth taking steps to eliminate or at least properly clean away these pore pluggers.

What happens when you get acne is that the stew of excess oil and dead skin cells building up in your pores attracts *p. acnes* bacteria. Using your pores as a snack bar, they multiply, producing inflammatory chemicals that send your immune system into overdrive. A surge of white blood cells starts waging war on the bacteria, leading to more inflammation and gunk, which together create sore, ugly lumps.

As for those lumps, they come in different guises that are helpful to be able to distinguish. First, **whiteheads**—those glossy white mushrooms that are all too easy to pop and aren't surrounded by inflamed red skin—aren't officially acne and quite easy to control with the regime described below.

The same goes for **blackheads**, which are basically whiteheads without a 'lid' on them and whose contents have oxidised and gone black.

Another example of lumps that aren't acne are **milia**, which look like tiny grains of rice under the skin and are not to be confused with a whitehead, as you can't pop them. They're mini-clumps of dead skin cells that got trapped deep under the skin and will eventually (think months or, unfortunately, years) travel upwards and exit your face. You can somewhat speed up the process by using a *salicylic-acid* gel as a daily exfoliating spot treatment. But if you really can't wait, see a dermatologist. They can quickly and safely remove milia with a sort of needle, but you'd be a fool to try that at home.

So, which bumps *are* acne? **Papules** are the mildest form. They're those small, raised bumps that don't look particularly inflamed (but are) and make your skin look lumpy. Then you've got **pustules**: sore spots that are red at the bottom bleeding into off-white at the top. **Nodules** are large, solid, red lumps that hurt and indicate severe clogging deep down in the skin. **Cysts** are as deep and painful, but these bastards are swollen and filled with pus.

Off-putting as they are, the most important thing to get over is the idea that spots must be nuked into oblivion with industrial-strength cleaning agents, scrubs and bactericides.

Yes, you need to clear out those pores and neutralise the snacking *p.acnes*, but you need to do it as carefully as possible. Inflaming your skin is just going to perpetuate the flaring-up cycle.

That's why any form of acne treatment—whether your breakouts are mild enough to treat by yourself or need a doctor's supervision and prescription medication—is helped by an anti-inflammatory skincare routine at its heart.

It also needs to involve a way of eating that's not making matters worse, and that means cutting out food that leaves your gut in an inflamed state. Skip Deliveroo, fried foods, refined carbs (white bread, cake, chips, crisps), sugar, sweets, soft drinks and alcohol—all of them make acne significantly worse. Eat fresh vegetables, whole grains, complete proteins (eggs, oily fish, meat—not sausages and kebabs) and anything fermented that delivers gut-calming friendly bacteria: pickles, sauerkraut, kombucha drinks, kimchi.

Dairy is an acne trigger for some (mainly because it contains hormones), but yogurt and kefir are a boon for acne sufferers because their fermentation has killed off milk's acne-triggering components and replaced them with friendly probiotic bacteria and anti-fungal properties.

BOTTOM LINE: AN ANTI-INFLAMMATORY APPROACH IS ESSENTIAL FOR FIGHTING ACNE

36 YOU CAN SUBDUE ACNE

(HOORAY!)

The common acne-tackling journey goes something like this:

> ... Buys lots of different 'miracle' products (on average ten or more) over the space of a few years or even months.
> ... Tries none of them for very long, or chops and changes between them.
> ... Finds nothing helps, and if anything does, it will for a few days only.
> ... The acne gets worse.
> ... Gives up and go to the doctor, who may say something like 'most people grow out of it'.

A far more promising acne-controlling regime goes as follows:

Buy a gentle, *sulphate*-free cleanser with *salicylic acid* in it and cleanse twice a day—not more. The last thing you want is *sulphates* stripping the protective acid mantle off of your skin and create low-level, sustained inflammation (you won't necessarily see it, but it's there). Do NOT use a bar soap—those are too aggressive and leave pore-clogging residue. The *salicylic acid* travels inside the pore lining, getting rid of the buildup in the pores as well as on the surface on the skin. It's also anti-inflammatory and antimicrobial, so it really is your best friend if you're battling spots.

Any cleanser texture is fine, but a wash-off gel or mousse probably feels best if your skin is quite oily. A thick cleansing balm is not a good idea as you want to stay away from anything too waxy or rich. If you use a lot of long-wear/twenty-four-hour/all-day (you get the picture) foundation, I'd double cleanse if I were you. Those foundations are causing a lot of skin trouble for people with a 'can't-be-bothered' attitude to cleansing.

You could follow with a *salicylic-acid* based toner, especially if you use a tissue-off cleanser. Make sure your toner (or ANY of your skincare, for that matter) hasn't got lots of *alcohol* or *witch hazel* (which is mostly *alcohol* and irritating tannins) in it; these will inflame skin and make your acne worse. The same goes for any kind of *fragrance* and *'cooling'* and *'tingly' essential oils* such as *menthol, lemon* or *eucalyptus*. They are rife in anti-spot skincare because we associate them with freshness and cleanliness, but they spell nothing but sensitising, inflammatory trouble for skin. Instead, look for calming ingredients such as *beta-glucan* and *panthenol* to give your skin a redness-reducing, purifying drink.

Dehydration leads to inflammation, so no matter how oily your skin feels, it needs moisture. You could choose a light moisturising lotion, a gel or 'sorbet' moisturiser or even a serum. Just don't try to 'dry up' oiliness. It can't be done and will make things worse.

Hyaluronic acid, glycerin, panthenol and *sorbitol* are the perfect oil-free hydrating agents for your skin. Certain *fatty acid*-rich oils (*jojoba* seed, *squalane* and *CBD*) can be great for acne as they fight inflammation while some kill *p.acnes* as well. But they need to be carefully dosed in a moisturiser, which will tend to be light, formulated for your skin type.

Apart from all the irritants described above, your moisturiser (as well as your cleanser *and* makeup) shouldn't have oils and waxes in it that are known to exacerbate clogged pores: *mineral oil* and *isopropyl myristate* are a bad choice, as are *coconut* and *palm oil*, and high levels of *cocoa* and *shea butter*.

Relying on products that say they are 'non-comedogenic' (non-pore clogging) is not enough. The term is somewhat outdated and backed by dodgy research. You're better off doing your INCI research on the back of the packaging, choosing a light-textured hydrator that doesn't feature the undesirables.

As for active ingredients in your serum or moisturiser: oil-regulating, anti-inflammatory *niacinamide* is always a brilliant addition and so are *salicylic* and *azelaic* acid. But I wouldn't use more than two acid-based products a day; you can easily overdo it. Any mention of anti-inflammatories and probiotics on the INCI list is a bonus.

And despite what you may have been led to believe, UV light makes acne worse, not better. In addition, the *salicylic* and other acids you use will make skin more sun-sensitive. So an SPF30 is essential, otherwise you are still making things worse.

It can be part of a well-formulated hydrator for oily skin or you can layer an SPF over serum; there are plenty of non-oily ones these days.

Alternatively, certain foundations *can* serve as your sunscreen (for daily use please, NOT on the beach). But they must be broad-spectrum, a minimum SPF30, and formulated not to clog pores, and applied so liberally (at least a third heaped teaspoon for just the face) that this is only worth a shot for fans of the full-on 'Instaface' look.

At night, spot-prone skin benefits from exfoliation with an acid (NEVER a scrub; it will inflame your spots). Because oily skin tends to have a lot of built-up dead cells loitering on the surface, this is one of the instances where you don't need to limit yourself to twice-weekly peels—just make sure not every other product in your regime is acid-based.

Avoid the more aggressive *AHA*'s such as *glycolic acid*. *Salicylic* and *azelaic acid*, both specialists at clearing out pores and calming skin, are the exfoliation acids for you (try either for a few weeks to see which suits you best).

There are even optimal percentages, based on scientific research not internet hyperbole. 2% *salicylic acid*, in a peel pad or as a leave-on serum you apply before bedtime, has been shown to be as effective against mild to moderate acne as prescription acne meds. 15-20% *azelaic acid* appears to be a close runner-up. As well as delivering a mild peel, it kills bacteria and inflammation deep inside the pores. It also inhibits melanin production, which is great for subduing post-inflammatory hyperpigmentation. The highest concentration you can buy without prescription is 10%, which still does a pretty impressive job of keeping breakouts under control, according to users I know who are managing their acne successfully.

Another overnight option is *retinol*, or an alternative

retinoid such as *retinaldehyde*. Retinol's acne-busting potential is well-documented, but so is its talent for irritation, which is why I would proceed with caution. If your acne is a major issue, you may want to go the pro route with this and ask guidance from a dermatologist.

Just a word of caution for those with black skin. Your safest option is *mandelic* acid. It has pore-clearing properties but it's the least likely to irritate, which is important for skins of colour that are hyper-susceptible to developing pigmented lesions when skin flares up. Check with a doctor if in doubt.

Combination skin

A note on combination skin, which is oily in some areas (often the t-zone) and dry in others (generally the cheeks). It can also manifest as skin that is oily all over, but is dehydrated (feeling tight) underneath. It's best to follow a calming regime for oily and spot-prone skin such as the one in this chapter, using a quenching, oil-free hydrator all over, but topped with a layer of richer moisturiser (look for ceramides and essential fatty acids) in the areas that get dry and flaky.

If your breakouts always happen in the same area, you can spot-target it with your peeling acid and leave the rest of your face alone. But if your spots tend to 'travel' all around face, just use the acid all over. Its exfoliating action has a preventative function as well as a spot-shrivelling one, which you want to make the most of if spots tend to 'surprise' you.

BOTTOM LINE: NIACINAMIDE, SALICYLIC AND AZELAIC ACID, RETINOL, HUMECTANTS AND CERAMIDES ARE THE HERO COSMETIC INGREDIENTS FOR OILY, SPOTTY SKIN

Cleansers, toners, serums, moisturisers whose ingredients I like:
CeraVe SA Smoothing Cleanser
Paula's Choice Skin-Balancing Pore-Reducing Toner
Garden of Wisdom (GOW) Salicylic Acid 2% (alcohol-
    free)
Garden of Wisdom (GOW) Azelaic Acid 10% Serum
The Ordinary Salicylic Acid 2% Masque

Medik8 Clarity Peptides Serum

Dermalogica AGE Bright Clearing Serum

La Roche-Posay Effaclar Duo Moisturiser

BareMinerals Complexion Rescue Tinted Hydrating Gel
    Cream SPF30

Dr Sam's Flawless Daily Sunscreen Broad Spectrum
    SPF50

37 DON'T HESITATE TO CALL IN AN ACNE PRO

Frustratingly, acne tends to be either over-treated—with the best of intentions but all the wrong aggressive, stripping products—or under-treated—where chronic acne, which really is a skin disease that benefits from medical-specialist attention, is waved away by general physicians (because it is not life-threatening) and suffered in silence by those affected. The bottom line is that, if a month's worth of a consistent pore-purifying, anti-inflammatory, barrier-restoring regime (as described in the previous section) doesn't begin to show improvements (remember, acne can be controlled but in most cases not 'cured'), instead of spending more money on products you should make an appointment with a specialist.

There are some really great facial therapists who

specialise in acne, but they can't prescribe medication so they can only do so much. Alternatively, there are dermatologists (medical doctors specialising in skin diseases) who can supply you with meds, but not all of them are interested in helping you look after your skin in the long run.

There are quite a few old-school derms out there who laugh in the face of skincare that's not classed as medicine. This is a shame as you don't want to just put medication on your skin, you want to treat it with nourishing and protective ceramides, antioxidants, and other skin-saviours for a full 360 degree skin-cure plus skin-care approach. The benefits are now well recognised by many in the medical profession.

To find someone who gets it, you might want to look out for a young-ish derm (make sure they are on the General Medical Council register as a fully qualified dermatologist; you can check on gmc-uk.org) who also offers aesthetic treatments and has a stated interest in skincare. Or you could look for a cosmetic dermatologist: these have a grounding in dermatology but a specialist interest in skincare. You may have to pay privately and that's expensive, but it could well be the best money you've ever spent.

Medical treatments for acne include *antibiotics*, certain *androgen*-suppressing birth control pills, *spironolactone* (another androgen blocker) and Roaccutane (*isotretinoin*), which is pretty much ingestible *retinoic acid* that shuts down your skin's oil production. All can be miraculous, or might not work at all. All have significant side effects and, often, they work only for as long as you take the pills.

So there is a real argument for combining meds with professional skincare, guidance and advice, or even for starting with a skincare routine tailored by your dermatologist and see if that's enough for you. If it doesn't work, they can combine things like prescription *retinoids* with potent cosmetics selected for you. The latter you are perfectly free to get by yourself. But, as we've seen, it's easy to overdo things and aggravate your skin condition. If you're battling a serious problem like acne, it's really worth paying money to have a pro guide you, monitor and tweak your progress.

Cosmetic dermatologists will often also do 'medical' facials, which can include things like acid peels, hydrodermabrasion (a sort of 'pore hoovering' with peeling serums), lymphatic drainage (to get rid of stagnant toxins) and LED light therapy. And they may look at your diet as well, to see if dairy, gluten and sugar are acne triggers for you.

The deep-cleansing or 'detoxifying' facials you find at your local beauty salon are not an option I would recommend. They can often be just an excuse to slap (too many) products on your face without much consideration of your individual skin's needs. The exception would be Dermalogica, who offer really good personalised acne-fighting treatments nationwide.

BOTTOM LINE: IF THE ACNE-QUELLING REGIME DESCRIBED IN THIS BOOK DOESN'T MAKE A DIFFERENCE, SEE A DERMATOLOGIST

38 SERUMS

A GREAT WAY TO APPLY PROBLEM-SOLVING ACTIVES

There is a lot of confusion about what a serum is and why you would need one if you already have a moisturiser. The way to explain it used to be simple. It's a concentrate of actives meant to tackle your 'specific' skin issues while your moisturiser is more of an all-purpose skin protectant cream. As a serum is much lighter in texture than a moisturising cream, you ought to put only a few drops on cleansed skin and apply your daily moisturiser over it.

But, as with almost any beauty product, where there once were clear definitions, the lines have rather blurred thanks to clever hybrid technologies and in some cases even cleverer marketing. So while the above holds true, a more elaborate way to describe modern-day serums is required.

Two things make a serum a serum, but they don't necessarily have to go together.

* *texture*. A serum is supposed to be a slightly viscous liquid that's designed to sink easily into skin. To add confusion, some brands produce serums in the shape of oils (sometimes called serum oils).

For an oil to be able to call itself a serum, it shouldn't just be easily absorbed but also have a lot of active ingredients, which brings us to the next point:

* *concentration*. A serum traditionally packs in a high concentration of skincare actives. It's meant to be the problem solver, the step in your skincare regime in which you precision-target your most pressing skin issue(s).

To mess with your mind, there are now plenty of serums whose sole purpose is to hydrate (their main INCI actives will be humectants such as *hyaluronic acid* and *glycerin* that attract water to the skin). These are more like über-light moisturisers for people who don't need or want anything oily or creamy on their face. The serum is, in fact, their moisturiser.

You may also come across light creamy lotions labelled as serums (to indicate they are highly concentrated and may still need a moisturiser on top) and boosters, which are concentrated doses of specific actives, a few drops of which can be worn under moisturiser or mixed with it (um, much like a regular serum).

Then some brands do double serums (bi-phase serum and oil which, once shaken up to mix the phases, infuses skin with serum that's immediately sealed in by the oil). Others (the Korean brands like this kind of stuff) do serum-in-cream formulations, which again aim to combine a serum and moisturising cream in one handy lightweight step. If you want a really potent serum, you won't find it in these creams, though. The 'serum' bit in most cases refers to an extra dose of hydration rather than an extra dose of actives.

There are serum masks, too—serum-drenched sheet masks meant to 'force-feed' a large amount of serum to the skin.

Yes, my mind boggles, too.

Though usually (but not always) more expensive than moisturising creams, serums are still your best investment if you have a particular issue you want to treat. So how do you incorporate a serum into your skincare routine?

The basic rule is that you apply it after cleansing (and after your toner or liquid exfoliator, if you use those), and before moisturising and/or applying SPF.

Here's what I would do with serums:

> No skin issues (signs of ageing, or sensitivity, or spots)? You don't need a serum; a moisturising cream or lotion is all you need after cleansing (remember, try out for the lightest texture that

still keeps you feel hydrated all day).

If my skin was oily and I didn't get on with oil-free moisturisers, I'd use a hydrating, oil-free serum instead of a moisturiser.

If my skin was normal to dry with 'issues' (lines, spots, pigmentation, dehydration), I'd layer a serum, or even serums if you're tackling multiple niggles (er, this is me), under a light moisturising cream or lotion. Going about things this way, you'll get far higher concentrations of actives that will actually penetrate to tackle the problem—they will have trouble doing that if you opt for one rich 'miracle cream' that promises to do it all.

If my skin was oily with 'issues', I'd layer my serums, including potentially a hydrating one, without a moisturiser on top. Despite what the internet says, most good products are formulated so that they won't 'clash' with actives in other products, so you needn't fret about one serum rendering another inactive. When it comes to super-potent retinol and ascorbic acid serums though, it is advised to use them separately: ascorbic for day, retinol for nighttime.

It goes without saying (I hope!) that an SPF remains imperative for daytime, either as part of your moisturiser or layered over the top as your very last product. Serums never have an SPF, so unfortunately you can't ever quite be a serum-only person, except perhaps on a grey day in the dead of winter in a forest. The good news is that your choice of light, oil-free SPFs is improving every year.

BOTTOM LINE: SERUMS ARE CONCENTRATED DOSES OF ACTIVES. THEY'RE YOUR BEST INVESTMENT IF YOU HAVE A PARTICULAR SKIN ISSUE YOU WANT TO ADDRESS.

Serums whose ingredients I like:

For spots: Garden of Wisdom (GOW) Salicylic Acid 2%

For lines: Niod Copper Amino Acid Serum 2:1

For pigmentation: Alumier MD Ever Active C&E+
     Peptides

Not-quite-a-serum serums whose ingredients I like:

Serum mask: Garnier Fresh Tissue Mask Fruit AHA Shot

Hydrating booster: Neutrogena Hydroboost
     Supercharged Booster

Oil serum hybrid: Glossier Futuredew

'Serum' oil: Kiehl's Midnight Recovery Serum

Bi-phase serum: Clarins Double Serum

39 FACE OILS

I love a face oil; I always have one on standby. Oils replenish dry skin and compromised barriers with lipids, and the light ones (*jojoba, squalane*) can actually help balance oily skin. Because they're made up of just plant oil and nothing else (although there are always a few rubbish impostors, of which more later), they are the purest and most effective 'natural' skincare available. With no need for additives like preservatives, emulsifiers and petrochemicals, they are suitable for the most sensitive skins and, due to lipid profiles similar to that of the skin, some may work at an impressively deep level. They've become so popular that every major skincare brand has had to add one to its product line-up. This is much to the brands' chagrin because you can't pad a face-oil formula out with filler ingredients such as water, silicones and mineral oil without causing a (social) media outcry; the profit margins on oils can be annoyingly (for the brands) low.

What they aren't on the whole, are miracle potions. They will not reverse ageing and make the rest of your 'non-natural' skincare routine redundant. These oils are often marketed as substitutes for powerful anti-ageing serums that moisturise to boot. It is true many naturally contain antioxidants, vitamins and even retinoic acid, but as you can never be sure in what concentrations (which you do know in products formulated with carefully dosed actives), it is uncertain what anti-ageing effect they will have. Many pricey ones are presented as 'unique' blends of oils with lots of different purposes. But the primary function of most oils is to provide essential fatty acids and antioxidants.

The main reason to choose one oil over another is its texture; some, like coconut and avocado, are far richer and 'oilier' than others such as hemp seed. So the drier your skin, the richer the oil you might like to use. Apart from potentially having a broader lipid profile to reflect the wide spectrum of lipids in your skin, a mix of different seed, nut and fruit oils isn't necessarily superior to a 'single source' oil like rosehip or jojoba. In fact, some of the blended products can be high in plant-derived but nonetheless processed vegetal oils such as *caprylic triglyceride* (which is great in your cleansing oil but not so much in a leave-on oil) with only small amounts of pure plant oils. It's a way to offer a 'natural' product while keeping the production costs down. Another thing you don't want to see snuck in your face oil are synthetic oils like *mineral oil* and *isopropyl myristate*.

You may have heard people (including some skin experts) claim that oils can make skin 'lazy', tricking it into thinking it's well-hydrated and so 'turning off' its ability to absorb and hold on to water. But this only holds true if you use tons of heavy creams and inert oils such as the above-mentioned mineral oil and isopropyl myristate on your face. They're a good sticking plaster in a dry-skin emergency (when you're climbing Mount Everest, as you do) but not a great long-term skin-hydrating strategy.

Finally, I'd avoid essential oils. Lots of people adore fragrant oils and many do have mood-balancing and even physiological benefits, but fragrance is a skin irritant, period. If you use a scented oil, accept the possibility that you could be sensitising your skin over time.

The way to look at a face oil is as an addition to your skincare routine, not the star of it. I add drops to my moisturiser or layer one over my serums whenever I feel particularly parched or dull or I gather my skin is in need of some healing. I've increasingly embraced the oils at the lightest end of the spectrum (*jojoba* and *squalane*) to avoid sudden mystery skin congestion. These two are said to be closest to our natural sebum so skin tends to be happy to see them. I also like *rosehip* which does have a little *retinoic acid* in it, so can be particularly healing.

Having said this, advances in biotechnology now allow for new types of oils with high levels of oil-soluble active ingredients that are a match for serums. However, they are still expensive and far and few between. But technology can move quickly and it is worth keeping an eye out for them.

It makes sense, as a good face oil is 100% plant-based, to heed terms such as 'organic' and 'single state' here, as it will guarantee the most active, effective and purest product. Extraction methods can make a great difference to the quality of your oil as well. If the packaging speaks of cold-pressing, CO_2 extraction, enzymatic extraction or steam distillation, you're likely on to a good one.

Quite a drawback of face oils especially if you pay good money for them, is that they deteriorate fast the moment you expose them to oxygen and light (i.e. open the bottle). It's best to keep a bottle (which should be opaque) tightly sealed, and in a cool, dry place. I know, these conditions are rather hard to stick to and I've seen my oils go off in less than a year. Beware of this happening. You can tell: like any oils in your kitchen, they will start to smell 'off' and rancid. And when they do, they create free radicals and become damaging rather than healing to the skin. I'd always go for the smallest bottle available. Skip the supersized ones.

BOTTOM LINE: OILS ARE A GREAT OCCASIONAL ADDITION TO YOUR REGIME BUT NOT AN ESSENTIAL ONE

Face oils whose ingredients I like:
Pai Rosehip BioRegenerate Oil
MV Skincare Pure Jojoba
Trilogy Very Gentle Restoring Oil
Kiehl's Cannabis Sativa Seed Oil Herbal Concentrate
Oio Brightening Facial Treatment Oil with Vitamin C

40 EYE CREAM...

I'm using an eye cream right now, because I've got eye wrinkles and I want to tackle them with a retinoid. But eye skin is thin and delicate and needs to be handled with even more care than the rest of your face, so it makes sense to try a formulation that is powerful but designed with those issues in mind.

And that's one of the very few reasons to use a separate eye cream. Overall, I believe you don't really need one, IF you are evangelical about your skincare basics. I'm referring to avoiding fragrance, alcohol, mineral oil and other irritants and occlusives in your face creams and serums, and using the lightest formulations that still keep your skin hydrated all day. Stick to that, and you can safely use any face product (except perhaps the richest face butters, which could leave you with puffy eyes) with hydrators, antioxidants, brightening agents and soothing ingredients around your eyes. If it's a cream, dab it on the 'orbital bone' that surrounds the eye socket and your potion will travel onto your lids all by itself, without over-saturating it. If it's a light serum, you can often cheekily slap it all over your eyes. Highly active and therefore potentially irritating ingredients such as retinol, AHA's or ascorbic acid (which can thicken skin and fight pigmentation, so tackling dark circles) can be too much for this area, though, so they should indeed only be delivered in a special eye formulation.

If your eyes are puffy, an eye cream that promises to solve this is going to disappoint you. Try a serum with calming, anti-inflammatory ingredients (green tea, azulene, allantoin, licorice), or just put two spoons in the fridge and plonk them on your eyes; it'll perk them up faster than any 'miracle' eye gel. Also, get an extra pillow (for added height) and a silk pillowcase: together, they'll minimise friction and help drainage, which goes a long way in combating angry, puffy eyes in the morning.

When it comes to SPF, which the eye area quite desperately needs, it's best to use a mineral formula (zinc oxide and titanium dioxide) only, because chemical sunscreens may irritate the skin here. If your sunscreen or sunscreen-containing moisturiser is chemical, you can use an undereye concealer with a high SPF instead, or resort to an SPF eye cream which is always physical.

BOTTOM LINE: IF YOU USE SKINCARE WITHOUT IRRITANTS AND HEAVY OCCLUSIVES, YOU WON'T NEED A SEPARATE EYE CREAM

Eye creams whose ingredients I like
SkinCeuticals Mineral Eye UV Defense SPF30
Neostrata Targeted Eye Cream 4PHA
Medik8 r-Retinoate Eye Serum

41 NIGHT CREAM...

While I'm at it, there aren't many reasons to get a night cream either. Obviously, SPF creams are only for daytime, while most retinoids and leave-on *AHAs* are meant exclusively for nighttime use. So that's where buying separate products makes sense. Beyond that, all the ingredients that regenerate, mop up damage and calm skin are just as helpful during the day as they are at night. If you insist on a night-time regime, instead of letting yourself be talked into buying the accompanying 'extra rich' or 'extra reparative' night cream when you buy a new moisturiser, use the opportunity to add a great active serum, like an all-purpose *niacinamide* or a deeply hydrating and regenerating *PHA*. Or use the night to build your lipid barrier with a natural face oil. Or if you use a non-SPF moisturiser (with a separate SPF layered on top during the day) just use that moisturiser at night as well. There is no reason to buy sub-standard products just because they're labelled for a time of day.

BOTTOM LINE: OPTIMISE SKIN'S NIGHTTIME REPAIR PROCESSES WITH A GREAT REGENERATIVE SERUM RATHER THAN SOME 'EXTRA RICH' NIGHT CREAM

42 MASKS

In the past few years, editor's beauty cupboards have seen an influx of masks. Hundreds upon hundreds of masks. Given that they are not an essential in any skincare regime, their popularity is a bit of a mystery beyond them looking 'hilarious' on Instagram before people got bored with that particular shtick. Masks were largely ignored (although always available) before that, so why are we now so into them?

Obviously, they are fun and seem like an affordable treat, and there's nothing wrong with that. But given that most of the time, they claim to have the benefits that you would normally get from a serum (hydrating, brightening, smoothing, purifying), they are also a damn cost-ineffective way of applying one, especially when we're talking sheet masks. These like to boast things like delivering 'an entire

15ml bottle of serum to the skin in one go'—but why would you want to do that if that amount of serum could last you a month? It must be because we believe two things: one, more is more and two, the sheet mask 'pushes' all that product right into skin for unrivalled results.

Well, more is not more; there's a reason why you only need a drop or two of your serum every day. It delivers the dosage of actives the skin can absorb in one go. Apply any additional drops or, er, the whole bottle, and it will just go to waste. As for that 'pushing in', the main reason any cosmetic gets properly absorbed is its formulation and the delivery system that is part of it. It has nothing to do with the mask, and any active ingredients such as brightening and peeling agents won't do their work more effectively or travel 'deeper' into the skin while trapped under it.

Yes, temporarily 'locking in' hydrating ingredients with an occlusive sheet mask will boost plumpness temporarily and leave skin beautifully glowy (and quite addictive that is, too), in the same way that oils do in a cream (water + oil). But your skin is not going to be permanently more moisturised because of it.

Applying a cream mask based on clay and /or charcoal regularly does make sense; these ingredients draw oil and impurities out of your pores and need some time to do it. Just make sure you remove clays before they dry up, despite the millions of pictures of photogenically cracked clay masks on Instagram. Once dry, they start sucking moisture out of your skin and dehydrate it. Not what you were after.

Another smart way to use masks is to apply a good acid (peeling) mask for the recommended time (ignore this at your peril as you could inflame skin) and follow it with a hydrating one. The peel *will* make your skin more permeable and ready to receive moisture and lipids at a deeper level, so this really does have the effect of a facial at a fraction of the price.

Still loving your sheet masks? Do the right thing and buy biodegradable ones made from things like 100% biocellulose, wood pulp or coconut fibre, or cotton, as the regular ones are the new microbeads/cotton buds/cleansing wipes, just adding to the Mount Everest of plastic pollution swirling around the oceans. I can't see the nylon and silicone ones being around much longer.

BOTTOM LINE: FACE MASKS ARE NOT THE ANSWER TO YOUR SKIN PRAYERS, BUT A PEELING MASK FOLLOWED BY A HYDRATING ONE MAKES FOR AN INSTANT FACIAL

Face masks I like
Alex Steinherr x Primark Maximum Moisture Supreme Sheet Mask
Trilogy Hydrating Jelly Mask
Clarins SOS Comfort Nourishing Balm Mask
Colbert MD Illumino Anti-Aging Brightening Mask
Zelens Transformer Instant Renewal Mask

43 SKINCARE HAS A RUNNING ORDER

Let's just suppose you're into using everything and the kitchen sink, as inspired by those Korean 12-steps. To be fair, even the Koreans are getting tired of these, but it's a good way to illustrate what ought to follow what. As a rule of thumb, it is all about texture: you should go from thin to thick.

Here is the order of application of products:

Oil-based cleanser: can be a cleansing oil, balm or milk. You're supposed to massage it into your skin to melt makeup and other oil-based filth, and rinse it off or use a moist cloth. Leaves a minimal amount of hydrating oil on skin.

Water-based cleanser: a foam or gel that breaks up dirt and pollution, and rinses off clean. If you want a more conditioned after-feel, you can switch the order of your cleansers.

Scrub: Don't scrub more than 2-3 times a week and choose a super-fine powder scrub or one with very smooth beads from natural sources like aloe. *Avoid if you're going to use an acid-based toner or serum.*

Toner: if it's a re-generative, hydrating toner, press into skin with your hands. If it's an acid-based toner or liquid exfoliant, apply with a cotton pad and avoid your eyes. Don't use both a scrub and a liquid exfoliant. If you really want to use an acid toner *and* a hydrating, regenerative toner, do it in that order, not the other way around.

Essence: this is a lot like a re-generative, hydrating toner, but tends to be a little more viscous (yet thinner than a serum). So applying it (with cotton wool or your fingers) only makes sense after an acid-based liquid exfoliant and not after a re-generative or hydrating toner.

Serum(s): if you use more than one (but stick to three max, think of your poor skin), the basic order is as follows. Exfoliating acid-based serums (like salicylic, azelaic or PHA) go first. If you've already used a liquid exfoliant, *don't* also use a leave-on exfoliant such as this. 'Problem-solving' active serums such as antioxidant, niacinamide or ascorbic acid serum go next. If you also use a hydrating hyaluronic acid (which, as you know, is not an exfoliating acid) serum, apply it last. Despite talk of deeply penetrating 'low-molecular weight' HA, these molecules in all but the most advanced of HA formulas tend to be quite large and could prevent other serums from penetrating.

(One caveat: because ascorbic acid is so unstable and pernickety, some experts advise not to DIY-combine it with potent exfoliating acid serums, and always using it directly on dry, cleansed skin, before other serum, to get the full benefit).

Sheet mask: if you want to build a sheet mask in your routine, it should go instead of a serum and before oil-based products.

On-the-spot treatment: if you've got a brewing localised spot (or two) and you haven't already used an all-over salicylic acid serum, dab a 2% salicylic acid gel or alternative spot buster on the blemish now. Try to avoid layering on any oil or moisturiser that follows (but do top it with sunscreen once your salicylic-acid gel has dried).

Oil: if you want to use a face oil, either massage it in before your moisturiser, instead of your moisturiser, or mixed in with your moisturiser

Moisturiser: choose the lightest one that keeps you hydrated all day (or none at all, if a hydrating serum is enough for you). If it has UV protection, make sure it's broad-spectrum and SPF30 or higher

Eye cream: use this if you don't want to use your moisturiser near your eyes, and make sure it has an SPF if you can't use your face SPF near your eyes

SPF: A separate sunscreen always goes on last. Sun protection isn't always easy to formulate with other actives in a moisturiser, so increasingly, consumers choose the best moisturiser for their skin and top it with a light SPF lotion. Some, I've discovered, mix it with their moisturiser: Please don't do that, it will adulterate the level of protection promised on the pack and harm your skin. So will putting on too little, which is anything less than a half (generously heaped) teaspoon for your face and neck.

Primer: Technically, this is makeup, meant to anchor your foundation—but some have a broad-spectrum SPF combined with texture-correcting properties (mattifying, illuminating) so could be used over moisturiser as an SPF-with-benefits.

BOTTOM LINE: IF IN DOUBT ABOUT THE ORDER OF YOUR PRODUCTS, GO FROM MOST LIQUID TO MOST RICH AND CREAMY

44 PACKAGING MATTERS

If your skincare contains anything active or fresh (most of the stuff you should want in your potions, frankly), it should come in packaging that will allow for the absolute minimum of light, oxygen or contamination. Yes, I know we can't help but be tickled by a pretty jar of 'precious unction' with a gorgeous-looking screw-on lid, but most products that can be exposed to the elements like that are not going to do much for you beyond moisturising your skin. Barrier builders with ceramides, prebiotics and niacinamide are also fairly oxidation-proof, as are a few antioxidants. But pretty much all other actives will oxidise (die, pretty much) within days of opening a pot.

The preservatives in your creams and serum are not going to stop this. They are just there to prevent moulds and spores from breeding in the pots that you are happily sticking your not-always-washed fingers in.

If you're going to invest in hard-working skincare, you want to see it in an opaque bottle or tube with a small opening or, preferably, an airless pump dispenser bottle or pot (one of those where you press the top down and a little product squirts out).

Put any lids back on after every use and don't expose your products to extreme heat or temperature changes. That includes not putting them in the fridge, which actually reduces a beauty product's lifespan. I hope you didn't order one of those 'mini beauty fridges' that became a sudden Insta-trend? Changes in colour or smell pretty much guarantee oxidation has taken place and you no longer want that product on your face.

Happily, the 'right' kind of packaging is fast becoming the norm among brands that are serious about their skincare. Pots and jars with lids have been disappearing from my in-crate at a rate of knots over the past year or two. True—it looks a bit basic on your 'dressing table' (if anyone today really has such a thing?), but what you lose in glamour, you gain in skin that actually visibly improves.

BOTTOM LINE: IF IT'S IN A JAR WITH A LID THAT COMES OFF, IT WON'T DO MUCH MORE THAN MOISTURISING

45 'ALL-NATURAL' IS BEST—NOT

I've watched the push for 'more natural' and/or 'cleaner' beauty products develop from a groundswell into a tsunami in half a decade, and it's brought many benefits. It's 'inspired' (you might say forced) mass-market brands to replace dirt-cheap and not particularly great ingredients, such as stripping sulphates and certain irritating petro-chemicals, with more skin-friendly ones. It's also prompted huge investment in clinical research of botanical actives, biotechnology and green chemistry, unearthing countless brilliant ingredients, delivery systems and extraction processes that are kinder to skin and kinder to the planet. And in the wake of a desire for more considerate potions has come a demand for more sustainable cultivation, packaging and production processes. It's all good stuff.

What is annoying, though, is the plainly wrong conclusion that skincare ought to be 'all-natural' to be safe and gentle, and that traditional cosmetics are mostly made up of 'toxic' chemicals that punch straight through to our bloodstream to slowly poison you. I always refer to a quote from Ren founder Rob Calcraft, pioneer of 'clean' or 'free-from' skincare: 'We leave out ingredients because we know of better, gentler, more effective alternatives, not because we think some will kill you or might turn a male fish into Lily Savage. If some agents were any more sinister than potential allergens, rest assured that the incredibly strict European safety regulations would outlaw them.' I can't put it any better. As for the assumption that natural ingredients are automatically less irritating to skin than synthetic ones—I know from personal experience that's a total fallacy. I've probably sustained more rashes and welts from 'natural' products over the course of my career than I have from 'synthetic' ones. I base my skincare choices not on whether they fall in one category or the other, but on a lack of potential allergens and irritants, which can appear in anything from cold-pressed natural plant juice to lab-made cold cream. The trend for 'natural' has brought great rewards but it is meaningless if a brand uses it as a guarantee for effectiveness and gentleness.

Here is an overview of the most popular marketing terms implying 'natural' credentials, along with what they really mean:

Natural
Means: Precisely nothing. Most products have some natural ingredients (such as, er, water). If a brand wants to big those up disproportionately, it can go right ahead.
Look for: Products stating a high percentage of natural ingredients (90%+). But check the 'non-natural' portion isn't just the sulphates and petro-chemicals you might not like.
Best in show: If your product is Natrue-certified. This international tag means the natural /and/ the small portion of man-made compounds sanctioned are strictly regulated, water can't be counted towards the percentage of naturals, and ecological and ethical production is enforced

Organic

Means: Very little. Put an organically farmed carrot in your cold cream and watch the money roll in; no legislation prevents you marketing it as an organic brand.

Look for: Only official certification guarantees plenty of organic ingredients and strict limitations on use and processing of ones that are not. Cosmebio, Ecocert and the American USDA are examples of international accreditations.

Best in show: The Soil Association Organic tag has long been the gold standard in the UK, requiring a minimum of 95% of the naturally grown ingredients in a cosmetic are organic. The rest has to be natural (things like water and minerals, which cannot be organic), with brands, producers, and processes routinely vetted for standards. Along with four other European organic certifiers, the Soil Association have created a European Harmonised Standard for organic beauty: if you see the words COSMOS Organic alongside the Soil Association logo or any other logos such as Ecocert, you know the product answers to the above requirements.

Free-from

Means: What you leave out of cosmetics, such as useless fillers and potential irritants (preservatives, emulsifiers, etc.), is more important than the amount of natural compounds you put in.

Look for: A long list of 'relevant' exclusions. Beware big 'free from' labels on products that exclude one or two 'nasties', but leave others in, such as shampoos that state they are gluten-free but use *sodium laureth sulphate* as their detergent. They're like 'fat-free' foods laden with sugar.

> *By 'relevant', I mean things that are usually found in the type of product in question and might not be the best choice for skin or hair. 'Gluten' is an irrelevant exclusion in cosmetics even for the small percentage of people with celiac disease, as it cannot be absorbed through the skin. 'Heavy metals' are irrelevant as an exclusion as they are illegal in cosmetics, so need not be mentioned in a special exclusion list. 'No sulphates' in a conditioner? Well, obvs: they are detergents and would not be found in a conditioner in the first place. Yet you see these things on bottles all the time, and it should make you think twice about the brand's morals and intentions.*

Best in show: Brands that state a hefty level of naturals AND a free-from list, like REN, Soaper

Duper and Yes To. After official natural certifica-
tions, it's the next best thing for knowing you're
getting value for your clean money.

Clean

Means: 'Free-from' by another name—but it sounds
more woke as it complements and piggybacks on
the 'clean eating' and 'clean living' ethos.

Look for: The 'Free-From' rules apply. There is no
clear evidence that 'halo' cosmetics that make a big
play about their 'fresh' ingredients, vegan ethos or
'detoxing' credentials will make you look better
than their dirty stop-out 'chemical' counterparts.
But, insist marketeers, the sense of 'holistic
wellbeing' they bring 'is really important to the
modern consumer.' That's you told.

Chemical-free

Means: Nothing. Ignores the fact that almost
everything in nature, including water, is a chemical.
May mean 'synthetic chemicals'—of which there
are many highly effective and non-toxic examples.
Could mean 'harsh chemicals' such as those the
free-from brigade eschews. Just guessing.

Look for: Don't bother.

Vegan

Means: Free from animal derivatives (honey, lanolin, cholesterol, carmine, etc. etc.). Most, but not all, vegan products are also cruelty-free. Many have ethical and natural standards, but it's entirely possible to make a vegan beauty product full of dubious synthetics and bottle it in single-use plastics. Bandwagoners who associate anything 'vegan' with health and superior environmental credentials, take note.

Look for: Vegan Society /and/ Leaping Bunny certification.

BOTTOM LINE: 'NATURAL' OR NATURAL-SOUNDING CREDENTIALS ARE NO GUARANTEE THAT A BEAUTY PRODUCT IS GENTLER OR BETTER FOR YOU

46 SKINCARE 'NASTIES'

After a good ten years of marketeers and 'experts' clamouring about 'nasties' in your cosmetics, you might be convinced they are full of toxic stuff. And after coming across the internet claim that '60% of everything you put on your skin ends up in the bloodstream' one too many times, you'd probably think they're attacking you from the outside in.

The truth is that the real absorption figure is about 2%. Skin is a pretty good barrier, not a sieve, and its main function is to keep stuff out. If it wasn't so good at it, cosmetic chemists wouldn't have to spend a fortune on research to get active ingredients to the right place in your skin. The small percentage of molecules that do make it into the blood steam are effectively metabolised, and whole government departments across the world monitor and regulate new agents and delivery systems, as well as constantly review guidelines on existing ones. When it comes to 'nasties', cosmetics laws, particularly in the EU, prevent the inclusion of anything at any level that isn't safe. There are only undesirable ingredients, and how undesirable these truly are depends on what bothers you, or doesn't, in terms of your skin and in terms of the environment.

Nonetheless, what's been very useful about the 'nasty' or 'undesirable' debate is that it's forced many new and even established brands not only to substitute slightly crappy ingredients for much more effective ones, but also to remove lots of 'filler' ingredients that were there to fill a pot at best, and at worst would prevent actives from doing anything useful for your skin. Think of how a bottle mostly full of water cancels out the effectiveness of the vitamin C in it, and how inert petroleum jelly seals in moisture but can also keep nourishing and regenerative ingredients from penetrating skin. Today, there are plenty of lovely products that are all killer, no filler, and while they are often a little more expensive due to the level of really good ingredients, they're still but a fraction of the price of some of the most notoriously expensive creams in glittering pots that the super-rich like to purchase from Harrods and Selfridges by the dozen. Those creams, too often, are high in fillers and bizarrely low in anything useful. But if the sparkle of a zirconia lid makes your skin look gorgeous, then the product must be worth it, I'm sure.

What are my 'undesirables'? I think I've already droned on about them. But as a round-up, I'll list the most widely named-and-shamed ones, and my personal opinion of them.

Sulphates
There are plenty of effective non-sulphate surfactants that won't strip your skin, scalp and hair but will still cut through grease. So why would you risk long—term irritation and dryness by using sulphates? Yes, SLS and SLES are the cheapest surfactants on the market, so if price is your main driver (perfectly understandably), you'll tolerate them in your shampoos and washes. Equally, if you require oodles of foam and a distinctly tight-skinned post-wash sensation to feel truly clean,

only sulphates will satisfy you. But consider two things. 1) non-sulphate cleansers and shampoos are now widely available from mass and retailer-own brands, at bargain prices. And 2) bigger bubbles have no greater cleansing ability, we've just been conditioned to associate foam with cleanliness. Whether your cleanser produces a bathful of bubbles or a modest amount of fine foam has no bearing on how well it removes dirt.

Sulphate-free bathroom bubbles I like
Love Beauty and Planet Shea Butter & Sandalwood
      Shower Gel
Yope Fresh Grass Natural Shampoo
Soaper Duper Clean & Juicy Passionfruit Body Wash

Silicones
They're plasticky-feeling polymers that form a layer to smooth frizz and bumpy-feeling skin, adding a flattering gloss to hair and a mattifying, imperfection-blurring finish to your face. Great! Problem is, products that feature silicones and not much else have a reputation for drying out and suffocating skin (leading to congestion) as well as weighing down and parching hair.

Modern silicones are certainly better than the ones of old (one or two huge 'first generation'-heavy silicone-based shampoo brands in the 1990s stood accused of making people's hair fall out). When well-formulated in a product, they are great at sealing in moisture without clogging pores, and some play a big role in the delivery of actives to the skin, so you probably use and like them more than you think you do.

The main accusation thrown at silicones, however, is that they are not biodegradable (the process whereby bacteria and other living creatures break these ingredients down). So, after use, the assumption goes, they'll be be swimming around in our waterways, along with our cotton buds and face wipes. Things are not quite as bad as that as silicones are, in fact, degradable: they will fall apart into their basic components—water, sand and carbon dioxide—in two years or so. Also, there are great strides in alternatives to silicones in cosmetics, so we may end up using far fewer of them in cosmetics. If you want to avoid them, most have *-methicone or -silixane* in their INCI name.

Products I like that feature silicones
Paula's Choice Water-Infusing Electrolyte Moisturizer
Niod Survival 30 PA+++
Glossier Priming Moisturizer Rich

Mineral oil and petroleum jelly

Dirt-cheap, good at sealing in water and almost universally non-irritating (there are exceptions— there always are). I wouldn't put it on my face if I had oily skin, and won't often choose it for my dry skin either, as I'd rather use oils with added nourishing benefits. I use it for body eczema and scaly skin conditions, although some research says the body can't metabolise the hydrocarbons in mineral oil, which can build up in in skin tissue if it enters the body through damaged skin. Other research, however, says mineral oil molecules (which are very large) cannot possibly penetrate even wounded skin. As long as regulatory bodies see no harm in mineral oil-based body creams, I see no need to avoid them in favour of expensive plant-butter based balms. We don't all have Gwyneth's budget.

Products I like that feature mineral oil
Embryolisse Lait-Crème Concentré Nourishing
    Moisturiser
La Roche-Posay Lipikar Baume AP+
Crème De La Mer The Moisturising Cream

Parabens

Ugh. Cosmetics industry insiders tacitly acknowledge that the reason every second product is now trumpeting 'paraben-free' is not necessity, but pressure from misguided consumers. A 2004 study that mentioned certain substances associated with parabens (a class of preservatives) had been found in breast-cancer tissue samples started a widespread internet panic that rapidly spread to consumers. Never mind that the research lead pointed out there was no evidence the parabens had caused the cancer. Or that parabens are some of the most exhaustively researched preservative agents. Alternatives had to be found, with interesting consequences.

I've already mentioned paraben-alternative *MI* (or *MIT*), which quickly caused an epidemic of eczema and has now been banned in leave-on cosmetics.

Then followed the scandal of mouldy cosmetics boasting 'natural' (and clearly not very effective) paraben alternatives. Also, cutting out this swathe of effective preservatives has forced the industry to rely on one or two options that are now used in everything. This, in turn, increases the risk of developing sensitivities due to constant exposure (it's often much better to use small amounts of a number of preservatives than a large-ish amount of just one). So basically, be careful what you get het up over.

Products I like that feature parabens:
.... Wow, there's hardly any today! Except for the entire barrier-boosting Curél skincare range, and the products are excellent.

PEG and PPG emulsifiers

These are petrochemical *glycols*, used to make ingredients blend and skin permeable, so the active ingredients can penetrate. But they are said to irritate a lot of skins. They also act as humectants, binding water to the skin. They can become problematic when used past their use-by date, when they can start to react with the elements and fellow ingredients and form carcinogens. 'Nitrosaminating agents' such as these are carefully controlled, but it's up to you to chuck them after the period-after-opening (PAO—look for the little jar symbol) expires. I routinely forget this because it seems a waste to throw out a half-full jar.

Brands without PEG/PPG I like:
.... Brands that specifically state they won't use petro-chemicals (ones with strong 'natural credentials such as Pai, REN and Trilogy) can generally be trusted not to contain these emulsifiers, but overall, they are very hard to avoid.

BOTTOM LINE: SKINCARE INGREDIENTS ARE INCREDIBLY STRICTLY REGULATED AND NONE ARE DANGEROUS WHEN USED AS DIRECTED

47 HOW TO SPY A GREAT PRODUCT FROM AN AVERAGE ONE

Judging from the questions I get, most people assume the price of skincare is a main indicator of how good it is. What price guarantees a product that works? Is cheap skincare inevitably rubbish? How can two seemingly identical products come at vastly different price points? Why should you pay a fortune when the doctor says a pot of cold cream is going to do as much for you as the expensive serum you just bought? Etc.

The fact is, price is no guide for quality in skincare, only your knowledge of ingredients and how your skin reacts to them is. You may, but your skin really doesn't, care how pretty the packaging is. Once you know the ingredients you're looking for and you spot them high up your INCI list as opposed to tucked somewhere near the bottom behind an endless line-up of *glycols* and *-cones*, you know you're onto a good candidate. And after the revolution that was The Ordinary, the skincare brand that blew up the industry by revealing what established actives really cost to produce (next to nothing) and selling them in simple formulas for a pittance, all bets are off. Good skincare is available at any price.

Aside from knowing what you want in your product, you need to recognise the rubbish you don't want. Or at least, need only in small amounts—that is, preferably not in the first half of your INCI list. These are not 'toxic' or 'dangerous' ingredients: all cosmetic ingredients are carefully controlled and anything used will be at levels that are proven safe. I'm talking fillers such as *petrolatum, silicones, alcohol,* and *isopropyl myristate.*

They all have a function in cosmetic formulas, but you don't want to see them making up the bulk of your facial products (in serums especially), with actives and plant oils bringing up the rear. At least not if you're going to pay big money, as is the case with a number of very famous, and famously expensive, brands. High levels of 'extracts' and Latin names (which refer to botanicals) give a good indication that your product is nourishing and active, as opposed to an inert layer on your skin that will merely temporarily prevent water loss.

A good trick for gauging whether you're getting a decent amount of actives is to look where they sit on the list in relation to preservatives (such as the very popular *phenoxyethanol*) and fragrance (*'parfum'* on the INCI list). The former is approved at concentrations up to 1%, while fragrance is rarely found in skincare at levels over 1%. That means that any skincare actives you find behind fragrance in particular is only present in minute concentrations. This can be justified in certain cases (we've seen, for example, that retinol is active at 0.1%, and so are quite a few botanicals, antioxidants, and other actives). But overall, when you see a significant number of ingredients you actually want for your skin, like plant oils, humectants, vitamin C and niacinamide, languishing behind *parfum*, *phenoxyethanol*, and other preservatives, you can be pretty sure you can do much better.

What you don't want to pay for either is packaging—not, at least, in the context of finding the best skincare at a decent price. You might adore the luxury experience, and find a cream in a gorgeous pot lifts your spirits because it is such a joy to use. And that's great, but if all that money spent on packaging and advertising had been spent on the contents of said (hopefully airless) pot, you'd have a spectacular formula instead of a half-decent moisturiser. So instead of packaging bells and whistles (and crystals and little spoons and metal-clad lids that weigh a tonne, which are environmentally not on), concentrate on packaging functionality: opaque, airless, hermetically seal-able, ie primarily directed at keeping active products fresh.

Other red flags: products (or their sales consultants) that go on about their 'iconic scent' or 'delicious melting texture' which are 'so important for the skincare experience'. No, they're not. They don't add anything to the effectiveness of the product (in the case of fragrance, they hamper it) and are an excuse to whack the price up (again, you might adore these things and happily pay for them—but this book is about learning to find out what your skin needs rather than what you like to look at). Oh, and when you get an undeniable whiff of alcohol when you apply a product (you'll know), think twice about buying it. It'll make up most of the product (check the INCI list for '*alcohol denat*' or *SD alcohol*' and it's likely in the first few ingredients) and that is never good for your skin. Alcohol is a cheap solvent and 'penetrating agent' for actives—but there are alternative methods for this without the drawbacks.

As for positives, independent clinical studies on the actives and formulas are always great, but really, they should be 'randomised, double-blind, placebo-controlled and peer-reviewed'. I won't get into what all that means, but that's the gold standard for findings that actually prove something and can't be spun and massaged by brands (and unsurprisingly, they're quite rare). Lesser 'scientific studies', *in vitro* studies (meaning done in a petri dish and not on living skin) and consumer trials—'91% of participants said their skin looked smoother' revealing in the fine-print that comprised only eleven participants—tend to be used for this rather enthusiastically and shouldn't be taken too seriously. As do brands that heavily rely on lab coats, pipettes and science chatter in their marketing without citing robust scientific evidence. A science-y message is no guarantee decent science found its way into the product.

Transparency and a brand's willingness to answer any questions openly, however, is always a great sign. It tends to mean a brand has nothing to hide, whether it presents itself as science-based, green, or simply as offering decent products at a fair price. All my favourite products are from brands with owners and formulators who are completely unfazed by my inexhaustible, detailed questions and will answer anything, even if they don't have the answer (which they will then set out to unearth). Of course, I'm lucky to have this kind of 'in' but I find that this type of transparency translates to the consumer 'experience' as well, especially for the smaller, digital-era brands, with loads of proper information online and social media access to the people with the real answers. In short, as with packaging, you're not looking for bells and whistles; you're looking for an up-front, open attitude that's focused on making an honest product that will make your skin radiate.

BOTTOM LINE: PRICE IS A VERY UNRELIABLE GUIDE FOR QUALITY IN SKINCARE

48 GREAT PRODUCTS CAN BE EXPENSIVE—BUT SHOULDN'T BE EXTORTIONATE

Nevertheless, I hear you ask, what should good skincare cost? Well, the higher in active and healthy ingredients and the more advanced the formula, the more you should be prepared to pay for it. If the feel of silicone or the richness of liquid paraffin works for your skin, that is great—I just don't want you to pay more than a fiver for your face cream (try a chemist's own brand or original Nivea in the blue pot), and not fifteen times that price for the equivalent by a prestige brand. When it comes to long-established actives like *hyaluronic acid*, *salicylic acid*, *niacinamide*, and *rosehip oil*, presented in simple formulas that need no tinkering on the part of the cosmetic chemist, you can get them all well under a tenner each, thanks to The Ordinary and copycat (but great) brands such as Garden of Wisdom and The Inkey List. You'll have to do your own mixing, matching and layering, which can sometimes be quite tricky.

But there are also well-formulated budget brands out there that take out the guesswork without charging a lot, especially if you're not blinded by what 'all-natural' or 'organic' credentials promise to do for you. Many pharmacy chains have great proprietary ranges with anything you need for healthy-skin maintenance under a tenner. For someone in their 20s, this should be enough. As for the big-name high street brands such as Olay, Garnier and l'Oreal, there's good, well-researched stuff to be found. But here, you will pay more for the brand names and marketing. To me, the 'French-pharmacy brands' such as La Roche Posay, Bioderma and Avène are more straightforward and better at leaving out potential irritants.

Once you venture into more corrective or anti-ageing serums and creams that are careful to leave out unnecessary stuff and have sophisticated formulas that tackle issues with a number of well-chosen actives and delivery systems, I think you shouldn't expect much from anything under £30 / $40. At the same time, you shouldn't pay much more than £80 / $100, either—and anything far over £100 / $130 is you being taken for a ride, with only a few exceptions. Breakthrough formulas and delivery systems, new (but proven) ingredients and potent blends that replace cheap fillers with nourishing alternatives cost money—but silly prices pay for silly packaging and celebrity ambassadors. My preference, always, is for products that don't bother with glossy marketing or 'beautiful' packaging, because I just don't want to pay for that. I'd rather see lots of lovely, skin-loving ingredients on the back of a simple box created by a thoughtful brand that only does skincare, and takes it seriously.

BOTTOM LINE: TRY TO SPEND YOUR MONEY ON WHAT'S IN THE BOTTLE, NOT WHAT THE BOTTLE LOOKS LIKE

49 LIFESTYLE

As if you didn't have enough potions to contend with, now there are scores of colourful new beauty supplements vying for your attention as well. Should you buy into them on top of all your educated and potentially costly skincare investments? Does topical skincare only really work in conjunction with 'internal' skincare, as some of these powders and jellies seem to slyly imply? Would it be clever to substitute a few beauty pills for a lengthy daily skincare regime?

Well, no, is the short answer to these questions. Supplements are a can of worms, and even more so when it comes to 'beauty' pills: these imply that you can take a supplement that takes care of a specific part of the body over all the other bits, and that is simply not going to happen. For one, your skin is your body's biggest organ, but the skin is the last to get any of the good stuff. Yes, a great nutritional balance featuring plenty of proteins, antioxidants, vitamins, and fibre for gut health is essential for great skin, but all of that should really come from the food you eat. There is no incontrovertible proof that the body accepts and metabolises many nutrients when they come in supplement form. And if it does, it's likely to be only when your body is in dire need and fighting a health issue that then leads to a skin problem.

Diseases linked to an imbalance in gut bacteria (such as irritable bowel syndrome) are closely related to skin inflammation and acne, so this is where a good probiotic supplement might help. There are also arguments to be made for a daily 2000 IU of vitamin D (the majority of people in the northern hemisphere is deficient, and vitamin D is essential for many bodily processes including the maintenance of healthy skin). A good multivitamin as well as an omega oil supplement are often recommended as well, even by supplement sceptics—as many people today don't get enough of these nutrients from their diet. But overall, caring for your skin from the inside out simply means replacing rubbish with nourishment. That means substituting nutrient-poor, processed, beige foods teeming with refined carbs and sugar (which is THE food-based skin fiend), with veg, wholegrains, (organic) proteins and good fats from nuts, seeds, olives, avocados and oily fish. Anything that nourishes healthy gut bacteria and aids optimum digestion (wholegrains, natural yogurt and any fermented foods, such as sauerkraut, pickles and kimchi) is good for the body and therefore good for the skin. As for drinking gallons of water 'to hydrate the skin'—yes, between one and two litres a day is wise for overall health (your body needs water for everything) but more water doesn't equate to better skin, despite what you may hear a model say (their skin comes courtesy of a decent diet, a lot of exercise, a lot of professional skin treatments, and the fact that they're 21).

As for exercise, it's a great helper to decent skin—it certainly is to mine. Forget the crystals, the jade rollers and the herbal tinctures. You don't often see an athlete with problem skin, and for good reason: the increased circulation, oxygen and nutrient supply, improved lymph and toxin drainage, exposure to fresh air and significant drop in stress and anxiety levels you get from moving your body are all major skin boosters. Any number of expensive facials and treatments try to achieve just that, but for a hefty price. You don't even need to go to the gym. Start walking everywhere, join a dance studio, take up yoga, or practice anything active that's has you working up a sweat and you get the benefits practically for free.

BOTTOM LINE: BASIC HEALTHY LIVING (FRESH FOODS, EXERCISE, RELAXING) IS THE BEST 'BEAUTY FROM THE INSIDE OUT' STRATEGY

50 INJECTABLES

At an over-the-top industry lunch not so long ago, I met someone whose age I couldn't begin to guess at. She looked much older than her way of speaking and expressions told me she was. She turned out to be twenty seven and she said she 'didn't use skincare' because injectables guaranteed she could party, smoke and sunbathe as much as she wanted while keeping her skin looking 'great.' What were the latest needle-based treatments she should try, though, she wanted to know? My friend next to me was cracking up as she knew the answer I was choking on. Not one, if you are well under thirty five. Unless you want to look like a prematurely aged waxen shop dummy.

It is the subject of another book, but Botox (an injectable neurotoxin that paralyses select muscles and so stops 'dynamic' wrinkles caused by facial expressions setting in) and fillers (gel-like synthetic substances that pad out and plump up bits of your face) are no substitute for skincare or help to prevent your skin from ageing.

Even the most ardent fan of botulinum toxin injections (there are various branded options) and fillers will tell you they do nothing for the actual quality of your skin—its translucency, clarity, texture, evenness in tone, lack of congestion. Yes, you can have a forehead like a bowling ball and cheeks of a hamster, but if your skin looks rough, dull or patchy, it will remain so if you don't look after it. As for age prevention: if you have any significant lines that bother you, botulinum toxin will get rid of them in a matter of days when they potentially appear at a later age. There is absolutely no need to 'prevent' them by freezing your face in time—this will lead, by the way, to muscle atrophy which can make your face visibly sag in later life.

There is the added fact that under your tight forehead and surprised eyebrows, your skin's elasticity, skin and bone density, facial fat distribution and even bone structure will continue to shift.

So while these treatments can somewhat halt the visible ravages of time and, if well done, can make ageing faces look less tired and indeed a little younger, they can't stop your face changing. So if you put too much stock in injectables, you can set yourself up for an increasingly desperate battle against nature. And we all know what that ends up looking like.

The injectables market is mushrooming and lots of interesting needle-based treatments and techniques that DO improve skin health are becoming widely available. Over time, these will perhaps eek out the more blatant and often regrettable 'work' we today so readily subject our faces to—although I wouldn't put money on it.

Clinical laser procedures pose a risk as well. Often presented as quite innocuous, lasers are in fact extremely powerful skin-resurfacing instruments that bring fresh but very vulnerable skin cells to the surface. This is helpful when you have a lot of cumulative sun damage (wrinkles, brown spots), or if you are fighting scars or serious acne. But there is growing concern that over-use of lasers over a

long period of time actually leads to increased pigmentation and faster skin aging. That is because the
virgin cells brought to the surface of the skin need
a serious level of protection from the elements
(SPF50, antioxidants) that tends to get forgotten
about, and also because too much 'controlled
damage' (which is what lasers cause in order to set
off a healing and therefore collagen-generating
response) eventually turns into, well, damage. If
you are over thirty five, proceed with caution rather
than abandon to address specific problems. If you
are under that age, getting a 'head start' on any anti-
ageing strategy is at best pointless and at worst
damaging. It's the same old refrain, and one I
would like to take my leave with: in beauty, less is
more.

BOTTOM LINE: INJECTABLES AND LASERS FOR ANTI-AGEING PURPOSES CAN BE GREAT FOR MATURE SKIN, BUT OVERALL ARE A BAD IDEA WHEN YOU'RE YOUNG

ACKNOWLEDGEMENTS

Special thanks go to my favourite beauty brains, for their real skin and skincare knowledge and their patience fielding my questions over the past twenty five years: Brandon Truaxe, Tom Mammone, Dr Dennis Gross, Daniel Maes, Dan Isaacs, Elliott Isaacs, Marie Drago, Marcia Kilgore, Véronique Delvigne, Nausheen Quereshi, Sarah Brown, Dr Marko Lens, Dr Nick Lowe, Rafaella Gregoris, Paula Begoun, Rob Calcraft, Shabir Daya, Debbie Thomas, Sally Penford, Dr. Sam Bunting, Noella Gabriel, Dr Sabrina Shah-Desai, Nicholas Travis, Dr Howard Murad, Dr Stefanie Williams, Fiona Brackenbury, Elisabeth Bouhadana, Dr Sarah Tonks, Marie-Hélene Laird, Art Pellegrino, Frauke Neuser, Pietro Simone, Dr Sophie Shotter, Kate Kerr, Dr Vicky Dondos, Abi Cleeve, Dr Wassim Taktouk, Dr Tracy Mountford.

Thanks for the love, Justin, papa, mama, Robert-Jan, Pepijn, Bauke and forever friends around the world. Thank you to all the UK beauty girls (and a few boys) on both sides of the fence—journos and prs—may we always remain the friendliest and most supportive industry you could hope to work in. Love to team Inspire and team Cosmo, past and present—especially the ones who suffered me as a permanently exasperated beauty boss: Cass, LC, Kate, Lucy, Jo, Kate, Philippa, Becci, Fi, Delphine: for God's sake! And thank you for the (loving) whippings-into-shape, Farrah and Louise: I love a teacher.

To my publisher, Martin, and to Allison, Savannah and Celia: what a joy it must have been (not) trying to edit an editor and frustrated sub. Thanks for the patience— we got there!

INDEX

Lightning Source UK Ltd.
Milton Keynes UK
UKHW011413120921
390444UK00003B/55